D0323350

An Introduction to Clinical Research

AN INTRODUCTION TO CLINICAL RESEARCH

Catherine DeAngelis, MD, MPH

WAGGONER LIBRARY
DISCARD

New York   Oxford
OXFORD UNIVERSITY PRESS
1990

MACKEY LIBRARY
TREVECCA NAZARENE COLLEGE

Oxford University Press

Oxford   New York   Toronto
Delhi   Bombay   Calcutta   Madras   Karachi
Petaling Jaya   Singapore   Hong Kong   Tokyo
Nairobi   Dar es Salaam   Cape Town
Melbourne   Auckland

and associated companies in
Berlin   Ibadan

Copyright © 1990 by Oxford University Press, Inc.

Published by Oxford University Press, Inc.,
200 Madison Avenue, New York, New York 10016

Oxford is a registered trademark of Oxford University Press

All rights reserved. No part of this publication may be reproduced,
stored in a retrieval system, or transmitted, in any form or by any means,
electronic, mechanical, photocopying, recording, or otherwise,
without the prior permission of Oxford University Press.

Library of Congress Cataloging-in-Publication Data
An introduction to clinical research
[edited by] Catherine DeAngelis.
p.   cm.   Includes bibliographical references.   ISBN 0-19-506249-3
1. Clinical medicine—Research—Methodology.
I. DeAngelis, Catherine, 1940–
[DNLM: 1. Research—methods.   W 20.5 I619]
R852.I58   1990 616'.0072—dc20   DNLM/DLC   for Library of Congress
89-22998   CIP

9 8 7 6 5 4 3 2 1

Printed in the United States of America
on acid-free paper

Preface

The purpose of this manual is to provide the reader with a practical, general approach to clinical research. Mostly, it is a primer for the novice researcher and is meant to stimulate clinicians who want to do clinical research. It is not meant to provide the reader with in depth information on all aspects of clinical research design, implementation, analysis, and reporting; rather, it is a resource for which more intensive instruction from other sources is advised at key points. The Suggested Readings sections at the end of each chapter contain pertinent references to address the problems that are beyond the scope of this text. An annotated bibliography at the end of the book covers special published articles and texts that can assist the reader for further, more comprehensive reading.

It is possible to conduct an important, simple clinical research project using the information contained in the text and some guidance from an experienced clinical researcher. After all, some of the most important discoveries in medicine were made and reported without the use of multivariate analysis or a mainframe computer. All research considered, Emerson was probably most correct when he said, "Nothing is more simple than greatness; indeed, to be simple is to be great." The reader, however, should not confuse "simple" with "easy." On the other hand, even though clinical research is not easy, it is exciting and can be habit forming.

This manual resulted from an idea of a former president (yours truly) of the Ambulatory Pediatric Association (APA) that turned into a special project. One of the APA's goals is to encourage and enhance clinical research. Hence, it seemed logical to assemble a group of experienced clinical researchers, who also taught clinical research methodology to others, to write this manual.

It might seem illogical for a committee to take on such a task, especially since it would be extremely difficult even for one knowledgeable and well-organized person to write it clearly. However, we did it anyway believing that there are real advantages to having 10 brains working rather than one. You will be the judge of how successful we have been.

Please note that while single authors are given credit for the various chapters, no fewer than four of us contributed extensively to each section by making suggestions for content, reorganization and, sometimes, rewriting.

The reader is cautioned that writing a manual on clinical research is somewhat analogous to trying to ride a bicycle while you are building it. For example, some of the terms used in Chapter 3 are explained more fully in Chapter 5, but you cannot really understand the contents of Chapter 5 without having read Chapter 3, and so on. First the manual should be read through in the order in which it is written. The various chapters can be used later to more fully understand some particular aspect of research.

Baltimore, Md.   C. DeA.
July 1989

Contents

Contributors, ix

Introduction, xi

1. The Scientific Method, Inference, and Validity of Research Findings, 3

   ANNE K. DUGGAN

   The Scientific Method, 3   Inference, 4   Validity, 11
   Suggested Readings, 13

2. The Question, 14

   JEFFREY A. WRIGHT

   The Question, 14   Consultants, 20   Literature Search, 21
   Suggested Readings, 24

3. Selection of Study Subjects, 25

   NEAL KAUFMAN

   Sample Selections, 25   Probability Sample Techniques, 26
   Nonprobability Sample Techniques, 28   Combinations of Probability
   and Nonprobability Samples, 31   Sample Size, 31   Attrition of Study
   Subjects, 34   Comparative Studies, 35   Suggested Readings, 37

4. Types of Research Models and Methods, 38

   LAWRENCE WISSOW AND JOHN PASCOE

   Classification of Study Design, 38   Choosing a Study Design, 39
   Descriptive Studies, 49   Cross-sectional and Ecologic Studies, 52
   Comparative Studies, 56   Suggested Readings, 72

5. Data Collection, Management, and Analysis, 75

MARIE MCCORMICK AND RICHARD C. WASSERMAN

Where to Start, 75   Selecting Instrument/Data Collection
Method, 78   Data Management Procedures, 89   Data Analysis, 94
Communication of Results, 106   Suggested Readings, 110

6. Pragmatics, 111

ANNE K. DUGGAN

Projecting Costs, 112   Minimizing Costs, 114   Funding, 115
Funding Sources, 116   Public Funding Sources, 119   Private
Funding Sources, 120   Identifying Potential Sources of Support, 121
Applying for Research Support, 123   Ethical Standards for Research
Involving Human Subjects, 126   Collaboration, 132   Suggested
Readings, 132

7. How to Read a Publication, 133

WILLIAM FELDMAN

How to Read a Medical Journal Article, 133   How to Read an
Article on Etiology or Causation of Disease, 134   How to Read a
Journal Article on Diagnosis, 136   How to Read an Article on
Prognosis, 137   How to Read an Article on Therapy, 139   How to
Read an Article on Screening, 141   Suggested Readings, 143

Annotated Bibliography, 144

JOHN PASCOE AND REBECCA HENRY

Glossary, 155

ALAIN JOFFE

Index, 161

Contributors

Catherine DeAngelis, M.D., M.P.H.
CMSC 2-124
The Johns Hopkins Hospital
600 N. Wolfe Street
Baltimore, MD 21205

Anne K. Duggan, Sc.D.
CMSC 144
The Johns Hopkins Hospital
600 N. Wolfe Street
Baltimore, MD 21205

William Feldman, M.D.
Children's Hospital of
    East Ontario
401 Smyth Road
Ottawa, Ontario K1H 8L1
Canada

Rebecca Henry, Ph.D.
Research and Development
Michigan State University
East Lansing, MI 48824

Alain Joffe, M.D., M.P.H.
Park 306
The Johns Hopkins Hospital
600 N. Wolfe Street
Baltimore, MD 21205

Neal Kaufman, M.D., M.P.H.
Harbor-UCLA Medical Center
1000 W. Carson

Cottage Street
Torrance, CA 90509

Marie McCormick, M.D., Sc.D.
Brighams and Women's Hospital
75 Francis Street
Boston, MA 02115

John Pascoe, M.D., M.P.H.
University of Wisconsin Hospital
600 Highland Avenue
Madison, WI 53792

Richard C. Wasserman, M.D., M.P.H.
University Pediatrics
1 South Prospect Street
Burlington, VT 05401

Lawrence Wissow, M.D., M.P.H.
CMSC 136
The Johns Hopkins Hospital
600 N. Wolfe Street
Baltimore, MD 21205

Jeffrey A. Wright, M.D.
Children's Hospital
4800 Sand Point Way N.E.
Seattle, WA 98105

Introduction

CATHERINE DeANGELIS

In many ways performing a clinical research project follows The Law of Inertia (i.e., a body at rest tends to stay at rest). As in physics, it requires a great deal of energy to overcome the inertia so that a clinical research study can be designed, implemented, analyzed, and reported. That energy requirement can be multiplied manyfold if the would be investigator does not know where to begin or begins at the wrong step and must retrace steps and do it again correctly.

Before embarking on a research project, the investigator must understand a variety of issues. Some of the basic pragmatics, such as grantsmanship, collaboration, human investigation committees, and resources, are discussed in Chapter 7. After these things have been considered, the investigator can begin to outline a clinical research project. Table I.1 provides an outline of the basic steps that should be followed in performing a clinical research project. The rest of this manual details each of these steps.

Study design is very much the center of clinical research methodology. Choosing the type of study design to be used is based on five considerations: (1) the question to be answered or hypothesis to be tested; (2) subjects; (3) methods of data acquisition; (4) type of data analysis; and (5) data reporting. Attention should be given to the following aspects of each consideration.

The Question

Choosing the question to be answered and ultimately the hypothesis to be tested is obviously the most important first step in research. Considerations should include the *importance of the question* (e.g.,

TABLE I.1.   Steps in Clinical Research

1. Develop a question engendered and/or motivated by experience.
2. State the question as a testable hypothesis (if you cannot do it, you still do not have a good question).
3. Search the literature to see if it has been answered totally or partially.
4. Revise (perhaps) the question and hypothesis based on your reading of the literature.
5. Determine what tools, materials, personnel, time, and so forth are necessary to obtain and analyze the data based on the variables you have chosen.
6. Given the preceding requirements, is the study feasible?
7. Revise (perhaps) the question and hypothesis and/or alter the variables according to your resources and time.
8. Choose the appropriate subjects (including controls, if appropriate) from whom data on the variables can be obtained.
9. Revise (perhaps) the question, hypothesis, and variables to match the subjects to whom you have access.
10. If you are still interested (and this is what separates the true clinical researchers from the dabblers), devise your methods to collect the data from the subjects.
11. Discuss your proposed study with a biostatican or someone experienced in clinical research.
12. Only now should you collect the data. Unfortunately, many novices begin this step much too soon thereby compromising the study's worth.
13. Analyze the data, with the help of a biostatistician.
14. Write it up for publication (this is what separates the academic from the nonacademic clinical researchers).
15. After it is accepted (and it might take several attempts), REJOICE, and take your spouse out to dinner. Better yet, let him or her take you out to dinner.

how big a burden is the illness?, is the answer to this question a key component of a larger question?, or how important is the answer to cost-containment in providing health services?). *What is the status of the area* (i.e., how much exploring is still needed) (is the researcher still fishing or stalking the game?) and how well supported is the hypothesis? *What are the characteristics of the phenomena involved in the question* (e.g., the incidence or prevalence of exposure or risk, the time span over which the phenomena evolve, the incidence or prevalence of the outcome)?

Is it ethical to conduct an experimental study to answer the question? That is, will some of the subjects be exposed to undue risk? *Is the research plan practical? Does the investigator have the necessary time and resources to implement?* Will the answer be unambiguous (i.e., is the question answerable by the research design chosen)? All of these issues and others are discussed in detail in Chapter 2.

Subjects

Unlike most bench research, clinical research cannot be performed without people, or subjects, as they usually are called in research studies. The *types and numbers* of subjects available are key in determining whether and how a study can be conducted. *How can the necessary subjects be enumerated* and *how can they become available for the study*? Very often collaboration between academic medical centers and private practitioners' offices are vital to address these issues. For example, general prevalence or incidence studies are virtually impossible if the only population available is a hospital-based clinic that is located in the heart of an inner city, poor neighborhood.

Chapter 3 provides an extensive discussion of these and other pertinent aspects of choosing subjects for study.

Data Acquisition

In many ways, acquisition of data is the heart of research design. The classic catalog of study designs used to acquire data are outlined in Table 4.1. There are at least four axes to be considered in choosing how to acquire data: (1) the investigators' and the subjects' orientations in time; (2) the investigators' and the subjects' orientations in the process; (3) description versus comparison of subjects; and (4) passive observation versus active experimentation to "manipulate" the subjects.

Orientation in Time

This relates to the number of points in time in which the subjects are observed and whether they are observed concurrently (i.e., the investigator and the subjects move forward together in time from the initiation of the study) or nonconcurrently (i.e., the investigator in the present time studies the outcome of subjects who have undergone a treatment or exposure in the past).

Orientation to the Process

This orientation relates to whether the study is prospective or retrospective. In *prospective* studies, the investigator starts by identifying subjects on the basis of risk, and then observes outcome at a later point. In *retrospective* studies, the investigator begins by identifying subjects on the basis of outcome and then looks back from that point. These two terms, and especially the first, are among the most frequently misunderstood in research.

Description versus Comparison of Subjects

Descriptive studies usually involve one population of subjects. Comparison studies involve contrasting among two or more populations. Either kind of study might be used to test a hypothesis, and both can provide valuable information. It would be wrong to denegrate the value of descriptive studies; as one of the contributors (L.W.) says, the attitude, "I compare, therefore I think," is simply wrong.

Observation versus Experimentation

In observation studies, investigators do not control the various factors involved; however, in experimentation studies, they do control them. The amount of control the investigator could have over assembling the study population and a possible comparison group, observing baseline characteristics, allocating and administering the intervention (if any), keeping the populations together, controlling the environment, and observing the outcome all need to be considered before choosing the type of study design and data acquisition.

These and other factors are discussed extensively in Chapter 4. The issues of collection instruments (i.e., questionnaires, chart review, etc.) and storage are discussed in Chapter 5.

Data Analysis

Chapter 7 provides the reader with a basic, do-it-yourself approach to data analysis, including an overview of the most commonly used statistical tests. It is important, however, to have a biostatician who will serve as a consultant for statistical analysis. It is essential to consult with the biostatician at the beginning to be sure that the planned statistical analysis is appropriate for the design.

Data Reporting

It is unfair for an investigator not to report study findings. It is unfair to patients and to other investigators who might benefit from the study, which should be one of the major goals of clinical research. It is also unfair to the investigators themselves because they can learn much from presenting their data to their peers. Frequently, suggestions are made that lead to much clearer and more pertinent results and future studies.

Usually, the reporting begins by presenting an abstracted version of the study to peers at a local, regional, or national meeting. It is wise *not* to follow the presentation ritual that takes place at some research meetings (i.e., lights out, projector on, read the abstract verbatum and presto: instant dozing of the audience). The odds are excellent that the presentation will be to a bleary-eyed audience who already have been shell-shocked by dozens of other short presentations.

The method of presentation is very important. This point is illustrated by the following anecdote. One day, while shaving, Mark Twain cut himself. He recited his entire vocabulary of swear words. His wife, hoping to stun him, repeated all the swear words. Then, Twain turned to her and said, "You have the words, my dear, but you don't know the tune."

Not everyone is a stage actor and it is not necessary to be in order to keep the audience's attention. Chapter 6 provides some helpful advice to assist in presentations.

Writing the abstract, first as a screening device for presentation and later to accompany the manuscript to be published, is often considered to be a monumental task. How can several months or years of work and reams of data sheets be explained in 250 words or less? Just remember that the story of the creation of the world was told in about 600 words. Chapter 6 provides a helpful outline of what an abstract should contain. The reader is also referred to any issue of *The Annuals of Internal Medicine* after 1986 for examples of very nicely outlined abstracts. The basic format is: study objective, type of design, setting, subjects, interventions, measurements, major results, and conclusions.

The ultimate reporting of data is the article published in a journal, preferably one that uses experts as referees. The process of submitting and responding to editors can be frustrating at times. Oliver Herford seems to be correct in his definition of a manuscript as "something submitted in haste and returned at leisure." The former should never occur; the latter frequently happens. Chapter 6 provides some guidance to assist investigators in having their study results published relatively quickly.

Real Life

It is rare for clinical investigators to spend 100 percent of their time in research. It can be argued that devoting little time to clinical or teaching responsibilities removes the investigator from the prime source of questions and possible methodologies.

At any rate, most effective (translate: relatively well-published) clinical investigators spend their research time working on several research projects simultaneously. That is, they might spend some time contemplating a question or developing a hypothesis; writing a research proposal for another project; analyzing or reviewing the analysis of data from a third project; and writing an abstract or manuscript on a fourth project. Of course, no sane person does all of these things on any given day, but over the course of a month or so, research time is usually divided among three or four different projects. This can be called the *varicella approach* (i.e., having a number of research "lesions" at different stages of development at any given time).

And that leads us to the final, yet probably the most important, factor in clinical research, *Time.* Serious clinical researchers who want a life-time academic career cannot perform reasonably without devoting at least 30–40 percent of their time to research. This does not include the nights and weekends that must be devoted to analyzing, corroborating, and writing.

On the other hand, full-time clinicians in private practice who want to make a significant contribution to clinical research can do so by collaborating with their partners and/or full-time faculty members at a near-by medical center. It is usually wisest for such investigators to work on one project at a time. Many excellent contributions to clinical research have been made by full-time private practitioners who have made vital observations and suggestions for the care of patients, which is, of course, the main objective of clinical research.

Some common reasons that clinicians in any setting give for getting involved in clinical research (and the traits they characterize) include wanting to find the answer to a question that occurs frequently (curiosity), wanting to share information and knowledge (generosity), and not believing that only bench researchers can contribute to medical knowledge (wisdom). Finally, and probably most importantly, there is a real joy in designing, implementing, analyzing, and reporting clinical research. This performing, just for the sake of performing, is probably what stimulates most of us to do clinical research.

We hope this manual will stimulate you to make contributions to the field of medical knowledge. There are few things more rewarding than finding an answer that will help someone and sharing it with others.

An Introduction to Clinical Research

1

The Scientific Method, Inference, and Validity of Research Findings

ANNE K. DUGGAN

The primary goal of research in general is to describe and explain reality. The potential value of a specific study is established by the relevance of the research question that motivates it. The ultimate worth of the study findings, however, is determined by the research methodology. Key aspects of research methodology include study design, selection of study subjects, definition of study variables, data collection techniques, data analysis, and interpretation of study results. Subsequent chapters in this manual describe each of these aspects in detail. This chapter sets the stage by exploring some key aspects of the scientific method, inference, and validity.

The Scientific Method: Relationship between Theory and Research

In the scientific method, the research process is not carried out in isolation. Rather, its purpose and methods spring from that which is already known, and its conclusions feed back into this reservoir of theory and knowledge. This relationship is illustrated in Figure 1.1.

Since research seeks to describe and explain reality, it begins by defining what is already known about the subject of interest. This is accomplished primarily through review and synthesis of the pertinent literature. A key product of this process is the development of one or more research questions. Beginning perhaps as a hunch, each question is carefully honed, and is expressed as one or more conceptual hypotheses that are grounded in theory.

The first step in testing the conceptual hypothesis is to develop a study design. While investigators are really interested in the hypothesized relationships of concepts, they must study them within the constraints imposed by the concrete world such a time, money, the availability of study subjects, and the state of the art of research methodology. The next step, therefore, is to rephrase the conceptual study hypotheses in operational form. This done, the study data are collected and analyzed.

The immediate product of data analysis is the study's empirical findings. The findings first are considered in terms of the study's operational hypotheses. They are then interpreted in terms of their larger meaning, as articulated by the conceptual hypotheses. This completes the cycle by advancing the limits of knowledge and theory.

Inference

As Figure 1.1 illustrates, scientific research begins with the larger world of theory and knowledge, moves from there to the more limited and controlled arena of the research itself, and then back to the larger world again. At the most basic level, the researcher attempts to describe and explain reality by (1) sampling a portion of it; (2) measuring characteristics of the portion sampled; (3) analyzing the measurements; and (4) interpreting the results. In the first two steps, the researcher moves away from the larger reality first by studying only a sample of it and second by studying only selected operationally defined characteristics of those sampled. In the last step, the researcher moves back to the larger world. This is accomplished by making inferences from the sample-specific study

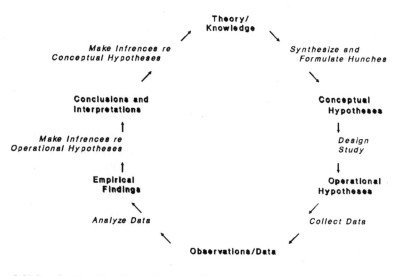

BOLD: **Content/product of research**
ITALICS: Process/stage of research

FIGURE 1.1. The Scientific Method.

SOURCE: D. G. Kleinbaum, L. L. Kupper, and H. Morgenstern, *Epidemiologic Research: Principals and Quantitative Methods* (New York: Van Nostrand Reinhold, 1982), p. 35.

measures of operationally defined variables to the hypothesized relationships of the theoretical constructs in the larger population of interest that are the real motivation for the research. The process involves four types of inference: statistical inference, causal inference, inference to constructs, and generalizability.

Statistical Inference

To illustrate the first step, suppose that an investigator is interested in the relationship between physician continuing medical education (CME) and quality of care in the United States. This could be studied, in an unnecessarily long and drawn-out way, by studying all physicians nationally. Alternatively, it could be accomplished by studying a carefully selected portion or sample of physicians. The methods used to define the population of physicians nationwide and to sample a portion of them are absolutely essential to the scientific integrity of this process.

In short, the sampling frame should be complete and the sampling method should be probabilistic. This means that the listing of members of the study population (the sampling frame) should include all individuals, and the study sample should be selected so that each individual in the population has a known probability of being selected. In the example, therefore, the researcher should select the most complete source of information for identifying physicians in the United States, followed by the selection of a probability sample using simple random sampling or one of the other probabilistic sampling methods described in Chapter 3.

After collecting data on CME and quality of care in the sample, the researcher would use descriptive statistics such as the sample mean and standard deviation to summarize the sample results. To continue with the illustration, the researcher might find that the range of CME in the previous year for the study sample is 0–50 hours, with a mean of 8.4 hours and a standard deviation of 5.1 hours.

After summarizing the sample findings with descriptive statistics, the researcher would use inferential statistics to make inferences from the sample findings to the larger population of physicians from which the sample was drawn. Inferential statistics assumes that the studied sample was drawn by probability methods. If a sample is not drawn by probability methods, it is not legitimate to infer from it to the larger population. If a probability sample has been drawn, it is legitimate to infer the sample findings to the larger population. Just as important, it is possible to know the risk of being wrong in doing so. Continuing with the example, inferential statistics allows the researcher to assess the certainty of the estimate of 8.4 hours of CME among physicians nationwide and the conclusion that among them, CME and quality of care are positively related.

Given a probability sample that allows making inferences to the population of interest, the sample size determines the certainty of the inferences. All other things being equal, the larger the sample size, the greater the certainty of inferences to the study population. In other words, as sample size increases, one can have greater confidence in the accuracy of inferences drawn from the sample to the study population. Thus, if the researcher in the example studies 500 randomly selected physicians, then that researcher can be more confident of the estimates of population CME levels and conclusions about the relationship between training and quality of care than if a random sample of only 100 physicians had been studied.

Like sampling procedures, necessary sample size should be determined as part of the study design process. Factors influencing the choice of sample size include the hypothesized sample findings and the desired level of confidence in making inferences to the study population. Procedures for determining sample size are discussed in Chapter 3. As will be repeated often in this manual, consultation with a biostatistician is invaluable for devising sampling strategies and determining necessary sample size.

Causal Inference

In the example given earlier, one of the researcher's aims is to draw conclusions about the relationship between physician CME and quality of care. While not stated explicitly, there is the implicit aim of drawing conclusions about whether CME influences or effects change in the level of quality of care provided. In other words, the study seeks to determine whether there is a causal relationship between CME and quality of care.

The study described in this example is observational, however, in that the investigator merely measures physician CME, quality of care, and their relationship. The researcher does not manipulate physician training in any way. By definition, observational designs provide relatively weak evidence of causation, primarily because they fail to allow the investigator to rule out other explanations other than causation for the association between the variables studied. In our example, even if training and quality of care are positively related, the relationship might well not be causal. Perhaps quality of care is a function of innate talent for or interest in patient care; furthermore, physicians with greater innate talent or interest are more likely to participate in CME. In this instance, the apparent relationship between CME and quality of care represents, at least in part, the causal relationship between innate talent or interest and both training and quality of care.

As an alternative to observational designs, experimental designs can provide much stronger support for inferring that the association or relationship between one variable and another is, in fact, causal. In an experimental or intervention study design, the investigator does not merely observe, but actually intervenes in the relationship between two variables. The investigator does this by controlling the independent variable, which is the variable that is hypothesized to produce change in the dependent variable, so called because its value depends on that of the independent variable.

In an experimental study of the impact of CME on quality of care, the investigator would assign physicians to groups receiving and not receiving CME, and compare the quality of care given by those in the two groups subsequent to the training. If physician group assignment is made by randomization, the design is a true experimental design. Probability theory provides a rationale for assuming that the two physician groups formed by randomization are equivalent or balanced with regard to all variables, such as innate talent, that might influence quality of care. The effects of these other variables on the dependent variable (quality of care) would also be balanced between the two groups. As a result, a difference in the dependent variable between physicians receiving and not receiving the intervention can be attributed to the intervention. For this reason, true experimental designs offer much stronger evidence that do observational designs for inferring causation.

While experimental designs permit causal inference, they often are neither feasible, ethical, nor desirable. In the example, there is an enormous difference between studying CME as sought out and completed by physicians in the "real world" and CME as provided in an experimental setting. Epidemiologic studies of the etiology and prognosis of disease preclude experimental manipulation of risk factors in humans. Health services researchers studying the public health impact of changes in health policy and the health care system rarely enjoy the luxury of controlling these changes.

Study design is the primary determinant of the legitimacy of making causal inferences. Within both broad categories of design, observational and experimental, there are many design variations, each with its own strengths and weaknesses in terms of inferring causation. These design variations, their distinguishing characteristics, primary uses, strengths, and weaknesses are the subject of Chapter 4.

Inference to Constructs

As noted at the beginning of this discussion of inference, the second step in the research process is to measure characteristics of the study sample. Reality dictates exactly what and how study data can be collected. While the researcher is really interested in theoretical constructs, these cannot be measured directly. Instead, the theoretical constructs must first be translated to operational definitions that actually specify the measurement procedures to be used.

To continue with the illustration, the research focus is the relationship between two concepts: physician CME and quality of care. These concepts cannot be measured directly. To study the relationship between these concepts, the researcher must first define them operationally. For example, the concept quality of care assumes the measurement of care in relation to some standard. Care might be operationally defined as physician response to questions on what actions to take in specified clinical situations. Another (more costly) way to measure care would be to assess the care documented in the medical records of patients treated by study physicians. A third (and much more costly) strategy would be to measure care by directly observing physicians in their patient encounters.

In addition to data source, another aspect of care that must operationally defined is its scope. While the research is probably concerned with overall care at the conceptual level, this would be extremely difficult to measure operationally. For this reason, the scope of care that is studied might be limited operationally to the process of care for one or more conditions, in patients within a specified age range, in visits occurring during a specified period of time.

Since quality of care implies some standard against which performance is measured, its operational definition must include specification of the standards that will be used to judge the observed care. For example, either implicit or explicit criteria could be used, with the latter drawn from existing standards of care, or developed by the researcher, or by special panels of experts, with or without input from patients.

Whatever the care and standards components of the operational definition, the theoretical concept of interest remains quality of care. Whether simply asking study physicians what they would do, reviewing their records to assess what they have recorded doing, or watching them to see what they do while being observed, the researcher is really interested in the care "normally" delivered outside of the study situation. Regardless of the nature or source of the standards used, the researcher is really interested in the "real" quality of the care delivered.

In some areas of research, the translation from theoretical construct to operational definition will be fairly straightforward. In research areas where more abstract concepts are studied, consultation with subspecialists might well be needed to identify or develop appropriate measures. Chapter 5 presents an overview of methodologic issues and strategies related to construct inference.

Generalizability: Inference to Other Settings

In interpreting study findings, the researcher is concerned with their ramifications for populations, places, and times outside the study situation. Generalizability is the extrapolation of findings from the specifics of the study setting to other settings. In observational research using probability sampling, the study sample is considered representative of the larger population from which it was drawn and so generalization of findings from the sample to its referent population is straightforward. Generalization to other places and times is not as simple, except insofar as the study sites and periods of observation were selected with representativeness in mind.

With experimental study designs, extrapolation from the study setting is more complex yet. As noted earlier, experimental study designs offer stronger evidence for causal inference than do observational study designs. This benefit is achieved by the control the investigator exerts over the intervention, the research setting, and the assignment of research subjects. Experimental manipulations, however, are deviations from the "real world." As a result, the same controls that strengthen causal inference weaken inferences to other populations, places, and times. The impact of sampling and of study design on generalizability are described in Chapters 3 and 4, respectively.

Validity

As noted at the beginning of this chapter, the primary goal of research is to describe and explain reality, and the potential value of a particular study is established by the relevance of its research question. Validity is the extent to which research findings correctly reflect and explain reality, and the degree to which the findings correctly answer the research question.

As the relevance of the research question increases, so too does the need for validity. Perhaps the most relevant research questions are also the most controversial, both because of their implications for policy and practice, and because they address areas where existing evidence is either scant or contradictory. To some extent, every research question worth answering is controversial, or there would be little need to launch a scientifically rigorous search for an answer.

Research findings are subject to controversy not only because of the controversial nature of relevant research questions, but also because of the role of inference in the scientific method. As explained earlier, the scientific method begins with the larger world of reality, moves to the rarefied environment of the study itself, and then back to the larger world. Statistical, causal, and construct inference, as well as generalizability, all involve estimating reality in the larger world from the experience of the study. Careful adherence to the scientific process increases the likelihood that such inferences are valid.

Cook and Campbell (1986) define four aspects of validity with regard to causal research that correspond to the four types of inference described earlier: statistical, internal, construct, and external. *Statistical validity* is the correctness of study conclusions regarding whether or not there is a relationship between two variables; that is, whether they covary. A study lacks statistical validity when it concludes there is no relationship between variables as they are operationally defined when in fact there is one, or when it concludes there is a relationship when in fact there is none. Such errors arise primarily from inadequate sample size and from improper use of statistical tests. The best strategy is to avoid such problems through careful determination of sample size and development of an analytic plan as part of study planning. The value of consultation with a biostatistician cannot be overemphasized.

Given that there is a relationship, *internal validity* is the correctness of research conclusions regarding whether the relationship is causal. If the investigator concludes that there is a relationship between two variables, then the next task will be to determine whether there is a causal relationship between them as they are operationally defined. Internal validity is jeopardized when the study design fails to control for factors that could enhance or mask the relationship between the hypothesized independent and dependent variables. Threats to internal validity can be minimized through prudent study design, as detailed in Chapter 4.

Given causal relationship, *construct validity* is the correctness of research conclusions regarding the larger referent cause and effect constructs that the variables studied were intended to represent. Up to this point, concern has been limited to the variables as operationally defined. As noted earlier, however, the researcher is interested in more generalized terms that have a referent in theory or in everyday abstract language. Construct validity refers to the truthfulness of generalizing study conclusions from operationally defined variables to these more generalized concepts. As described in Chapter 5, the use of valid and reliable measures is prerequisite to the construct validity of research findings.

Finally, given a causal relationship between the intended referent constructs, *external validity* is the correctness of generalizing the research findings to other persons, settings, and times. The researcher seeks not only to generalize from operationally defined variables to constructs, but also from a particular study sample to a larger population and possibly to other populations, settings, and times as well. External validity refers to the truthfulness of making such inferences. Strategies for maximizing external validity relate both to sampling (Chapter 3) and study design (Chapter 4).

Conclusion

In summary, the scientific process involves making inferences from the specifics of the study situation to the larger world. The value of research depends on the validity of such inferences. The researcher's choice of methods determines the validity of study inferences. The chapters that follow explain the strengths and weaknesses of the choices available.

Suggested Readings

Cook, T. D., and Campbell, D. T. *Quasi-Experimentation: Design and Analysis Issues for Field Settings.* Boston: Houghton Mifflin Company, 1979.
See Chapter 1: Causal Inference and the Language of Experimentation.

Kerlinger, F. N. *Foundations of Behavioral Research.* 3rd ed. New York: Holt, Rinehart and Winston, 1986.
See Chapter 1: Science and *Scientific Approach.*

Kidder, L. H. *Selltiz, Wrightsman and Cook's Research Methods in Social Relations.* New York: Holt, Rinehart and Winston, 1981.
See Chapter 1: Exploring the Social World.

Kleinbaum, D. G.; Kupper, L. L.; and Morgenstern, H. *Epidemiologic Methods: Principles and Quantitative Methods.* New York: Van Nostrand Reinhold, 1982.
See Chapter 1: Key Issues in Epidemiologic Research—An Overview.

2

The Question

JEFFREY A. WRIGHT

The Question

"To be or not to be . . . ?", that is not a good clinical research question. Ask any researcher who has tried to answer it. The key to success in clinical research is to frame a relevant question that is answerable with the subjects, time, money, staff, etc., available and the willingess of the researcher to see it through.

The prelude to research is the generation of a specific type of question. Development of a research project involves examining that question and distilling it to a precise, testable statement (hypothesis). The type of question essentially determines the method of research to be used and the type of result achieved. The initial question is often simple and general. It generates a trail of other questions such as: How could that question be answered?; What kind of study would provide the answer?; What tools can be developed to collect the data?; How much information needs to be collected to supply valid results?; What statistical methods are available to evaluate these data?; What are the possible answers (outcomes) to the question?; and Will these answers be useful? All of this leads to the ultimate question: So what? If the research is not excited about the answer to this final question, the study is probably not worth the effort. Start over again.

The process of answering the questions mentioned earlier refines the study so that clear direction is given for further investigation. Questions arise from an individual's native curiosity, and they can be stimulated by exposure to patient care, reading the publications of others, and by discussion among colleagues. Whenever critical thought is applied, questions will arise. The problem is usually that there are too many questions, rather than not enough. Some questions are worth trying to answer, others are not. The difference depends on the worth of the result compared to the difficulty and cost of obtaining it. The range of questions is infinite, but the methods of deriving a vlid answer are limited. Often, availability of resources and time dictates what kinds of questions can be answered.

It is important to avoid asking too broad a question or too many questions at once, since no single study can provide all the information desired. Sometimes exploration of a question will raise many new issues and further questions, but it can also eliminate extraneous facets involved in the basic question. It is important to narrow the research question to avoid pursuing many irrelevant or unimportant channels. Conversely, a question that is too narrow will not allow results that are of interest to many other persons or that can be applied to a more general population.

For example, the researcher might wish to know the effectiveness of "Ommicillin" against infections. The question, Is "Ommicillin" effective in treating infections?, is much too broad to be answered. The researcher must decide on which issues are important. These include what organisms, what type of infections (such as pneumonia, otitis media, cellititis), what age group, what dosage, and so forth, are to be considered. On the other hand, the question, Is "Ommicillin" effective against *X. rariformis* infections in 98-year-old albinos?, would not be of much interest to most clinicians. Furthermore, even though the latter question has a yes/no answer and is therefore relatively easy to answer statistically, the study population might be impossible to find. While these examples might seem obvious, they make a point that must be remembered before embarking on any study. Attention to detail in choosing an appropriate and clinically relevant question will greatly reduce the chance that the study results will be ambiguous or not useful because the wrong question was asked.

Factors that might possibly uncover or, of themselves, be constraints to development of a reasonable, answerable research question are:

1. Literature review
2. Time
3. Cost of materials, tests, assistants, etc.
4. Sufficient number and types of subjects
5. Ability to gather and store data
6. Critical mass of colleagues interested in clinical research
7. Ethical issues.

The following are some general suggestions for generating a reasonable question and developing a working hypothesis. The various methods available to answer the question are discussed in detail in Chapter 4, but it is vital to understand that it is the question that determines the course of subsequent study.

Generate an Idea

Several factors are necessary to generate creative ideas. Most importantly, a proper mental attitude including curiosity, energy, and a healthy dose of skepticism is needed. Also, the investigator must be willing to accept responsibility for finding the answer while honestly adhering to the rigors of the scientific method.

Proper environmental conditions must also be present. An atmosphere of questioning and discussion, with feedback and critique from colleagues, including someone with a sound knowledge of biostatistics, is helpful to view problems from different perspectives. Some institutions form research clubs or have a regular in-house research seminar where investigators share work in progress or practice presentations. An institutional human investigation review board can also provide good suggestions for modification of study methods. Access to library services is necessary to find background material.

Identify a Simple Question

The first step in identifying a simple question is to begin with a *direct question* that usually involves a high level of abstraction. In other words, it is a broad general question such as: What factors lead to otitis media in children?

Modify the Question

The next question is to distill the question to form a specific, testable hypothesis. Hypothesis testing, which is a method for choosing between the null hypothesis and alternative hypothesis, is discussed later. A hypothesis is a statement that proposes a relationship between specific *factors* or variables. The factor is an attribute or characteristic of the person, place, or time that is in the question. The factors involving persons can include age, weight, sex, race, and income. Place refers to physical location such as day care center, home, bathrooms, or more abstract places such as rural or urban. Time factors are minutes, hours, months, and years or seasons, quarters, semesters, and so forth.

In the distilling phase the question begins to define specific factors that might be studied. They can be descriptive: What is the otitis media rate in winter?, or seek to find a difference: Is there a difference between otitis media rates in the suburbs compared to urban areas?, or explore some type of relationship: As maternal education level varies, what happens to the number of otitis media follow-up visits?.

The factors must be objective and measurable. For example the question, Are male physicians better than female physicians in diagnosing otitis media?, is not a good question because "better" is neither objective nor measurable.

Except for descriptive studies there must be at least two or more factors in a question. The question, Do young infants have more episodes of otitis media?, is not a good question. It begs for another question, Than whom? The only factor in the question is "episodes of otitis media." The question could be rewritten as, Do children under one year of age have more episodes of otitis media than those older than one year of age? Through the addition of the factor, age, this question has two variables and can be studied.

Form a Hypothesis

The next step is to form an hypothesis or hypotheses from the question. The hypothesis is the researcher's prediction of the results. It can be stated logically, "if X, then Y" thus linking the data to theory. Using the hypothesis as a testable comparison between two responses, the research problem can be distilled into its components.

There are two basic types of hypotheses used: the *null hypothesis* and the *alternative hypothesis*. The null hypothesis predicts no difference between comparison groups, while the alternative hypothesis predicts that there is a difference and might also indicate the direction of that difference. The proper statement of the hypothesis is critical, as it clarifies the question and influences the choice of statistical tests that can be used in analyzing the results. An example of the null hypothesis is: There is no month to month variation in the prevalence of otitis media. An alternative hypothesis is: Otitis media is more prevalent in the winter than in other seasons.

Questions may be simple or complex. A simple question may relate two factors, while a complex question relates many factors. The number of factors will determine the type of study and the statistical analysis of the results. This is discussed further in subsequent chapters.

Perhaps the best way to practice developing legitimate, answerable research questions and hypotheses is to write down as many questions about a topic as is possible. Each written question is refined to a null or directional difference statement. This includes consideration of all the factors needed to gather appropriate data and the various factors that need to be controlled because they might influence the outcome.

Measures

To translate the terms of the question into procedures, operational definitions need to be developed. This identifies the factors to study or to control. In the otitis example stated earlier, an operational statement can be made such as: A group of children equally balanced in numbers by age, sex, and race are followed for 1 year with the number of episodes of otitis media recorded. The number of episodes per child per month are tallied. This details the operation, or data collection planned, and shows how the rate of otitis in winter will be computed.

After the hypothesis is well defined, the factors to be measured need further analysis. This involves first the identification of the *criterion measure*, which is also called the *dependent variable*. This is the outcome factor to be measured. For example, in a study to determine the effects of salt intake on hypertension, the blood pressure is the dependent variable. Selection of the dependent variable may be based on previous research or by the experience, judgment, and intuition of the researcher, which suggest that a logical relationship exists.

Because some factors cannot be measured directly, their existence must be inferred from measurements of certain attributes that are observable and are believed to indicate something about the factor. It becomes important to make sure that the dependent variable actually reflects some attribute of the factor. For example: A study is proposed to test the effectiveness of an educational program given to postpartum mothers. The hypothesis is: Educated mothers make fewer neonatal physician visits. The mothers are divided into two groups, the *control* group, which receives traditional postpartum education, and the *test* group, which receives the intervention program.

In this example the dependent variable is the number of neonatal visits. The factor that the researcher is really interested in is the effect of learning on neonatal visits, but that is much more difficult to measure directly. The assumption is that the change in neonatal visit behavior is related to the learning received through education. The performance (visits) is an attribute of learning. Some difference in behavior may be due to the perceptions of the mothers, and there might be other factors not considered or controlled that are responsible for the behavior. In many studies it is assumed that these factors will "average out" in the study and the control groups providing the group subjects are randomly assigned and comprise a sufficient number. This concept is discussed more fully in Chapter 4.

Selection of the dependent variable may be based on previous research or by the experience, judgment, and intuition of the researcher, which suggests that a logical relationship exists. Other considerations include the selection of the most efficiently communicative unit (inches versus rods) and the sensitivity of the measure.

Independent variables are the measurable factors that may affect the dependent variable. In experimental studies the independent variable is the factor (the intervention or treatment) that is hypothesized to influence outcomes. In the previously cited example, the independent variable is the educational program.

Stated another way, by manipulating the independent variable (the intervention), the researcher observes the effect on the dependent variable (the outcome). For example, in a study of hypertension in which the effectiveness of two medications are compared, the different medications are the independent variables, and blood pressure is the dependent variable.

The most important concept in research question development is that the process is circular. The question determines the type of study and the statistical methods used. Likewise the availability of an appropriate method will determine whether the question is answerable. This leads to this simple rule: The statistical methods needed should be arranged *before* the study begins, not after data collection has started.

Consultants

The ultimate success of a project depends on the planning that occurs prior to data collection. An important concept to remember, at this point, is that for a study to reach completion, the question must be answerable by a reasonable method. This includes considering whether the cost for using a particular method is justified in view of the expected benefits gained from the answer. Also, practical issues need to be examined, such as whether the perceived inconvenience, cost, time, and so forth, of performing the project and analyzing data make completion unduly difficult or not feasible. This applies to the investigator, to the subjects, and possibly to the investigator's colleagues. A project of long duration should only be started by those who expect to be around to finish it.

It is a good idea to have colleagues play devil's advocate with the project. For example, the investigator might consider that certain noncontrollable factors assigned (such as mother's perceptions) would average out in randomly assigned study and control groups. A colleague might not agree and present conceivable arguments to support his or her view; therefore, the investigator might well decide on a different study method based on other's input.

Finally, and it cannot be overstated, statistical consultation must be available to help analyze the results to support the validity of the study. The statistical consultation needed should be arranged *before* the study begins, not after data collection has started! Statistical factors may restrict the question that can be asked. Some questions that seem very important to our understanding of the world may need to wait for the proper ingredients to be present before they can be answered.

Literature Search

Even though the literature might have helped to generate the question, after developing the specific question for research it is important to search the literature to define in detail what is known about the subject. Has the study already been done? Are there related studies that would complement the current investigation? Reading published protocols might help outline investigative procedures. These are usually found in the methods section of an article. The discussion section may disclose other facets such as problems encountered with the study and suggestions for future research areas. This may lead to rethinking the experimental design.

Traditionally, literature searches involved reviewing lists of references at the ends of articles on a particular subject and periodic meetings or conversations with colleagues engaged in similar research. As the number of investigators increases and the areas of research become more specialized, it is more difficult to keep current in a particular field. This has led to the development of agencies that gather and catalog references. Probably the source most familiar to clinicians is *The Index Medicus*, a printed form of the National Library of Medicine Bibliography. It contains references from more than 3,000 journals published in the United States and internationally and is usually readily available in medical libraries. The advantage of using this index is that it allows the reader to pursue many key words that may lead to trails of associated subjects.

With the information explosion of the 1980s, computer data base storage systems become available. The United States National Library of Medicine has developed 16 different data bases that contain about 6 million references. This is (Medical Literature Analysis and Retrieval System or MEDLARS). One of these data bases is called MEDLINE. It is a bibliographic file of articles, and it is the most comprehensive, economical and widely used system. A number of vendors offer access to MEDLINE alone or in addition to other services. The price of using the service varies with the vendor, with some offering discounts for evening or weekend use. Some have subscription fees and all charge proportionately to the number of minutes connected by computer or terminal over telephone lines (online) to the service. Some services can be directly accessed by a personal computer. Some vendors sell or lease terminals directly connected to their service while others must be accessed through a connecting service that allows users from a region to link to a central node that has direct access to the system. These are called *packet switching networks* and include companies such as GTE, Telenet, and Uninet. The advantage of a direct terminal is in ease of operation. The advantage of a computer is that search criteria may be prepared before calling the service (offline), and bulk information may be transferred to the computer (downloaded) and examined at leisure. Both of these maneuvers save on costs.

The main advantage in using computer searches is in the rapidity of information retrieval and thoroughness of the search, if done properly. When considering the cost it is important to weigh the investigator's time in travel to the library and manual searching against the quick, but charged time, by computer.

The minimal equipment needed is a personal computer with two disk drives, a communications program (some are available free), and a modem that connects the computer to a telephone line. It is nice to have a printer and extra storage such as a hard disk, but these are not essential. A number of vendors also offer software (computer programs) that simplify the search process.

The vendors offering access to information data bases vary primarily in ease of accessing the file listings and cost. All of the systems require a certain vocabulary or computer literacy. Of course, searches can be performed by medical librarians, but more systems are now user friendly and clinicians can do their own searches using simple steps. The advantage of the investigator personally doing the search is greater ability to narrow the references quickly by modifying the search strategy online.

A recently developed alternative to online searches is the CD ROM. This is a compact laser disk (CD) on which is stored a mass of MEDLINE data in a "read only" format (ROM). These are usually updated annually so the most recent articles may not be present, but past publications are available. This disk may be purchased by a library. Searches can be done using a disk reading terminal. The advantage of this method is that after the initial investment for the reader and disk there are no additional charges for search time, which saves money in institutions that perform many searches.

BRS/Saunders offers MEDLINE in addition to 15 journals and 25 books now available in full-text form. Mead Data Central has developed a medical full-text service called MEDIS that has recently added *American Journal of Diseases of Children* to its listings of 49 journals. MEDLINE is also available through MEDIS. The American Medical Association provides a multipurpose information service that includes MEDLINE and MINET, full-text drug and disease descriptions, CME programs, a medical news service, and electronic mail service. DIALOG has the widest range of service and offers access to hundreds of data bases including MEDLINE and SCISEARCH, a data base of all the scientific and technological journals. It has access to an encyclopedia, an electronic mail service, and even a data base of data bases!

The least expensive access to MEDLINE is NLM, a service directly from the National Library of Medicine, but it is not the easiest to use. The easiest is probably Paperchase, which is now available through Compuserve, a popular consumer computer system featuring online banking, computer clubs, airline reservations, stock market quotes, and an online shopping mall (unfortunately it does not do windows!). Paperchase is also one of the most expensive services. It is important to remember that this industry is changing rapidly, and this information will become outdated quickly. The following table provides telephone numbers of some services available now; however, remember that this is a rapidly expanding and constantly changing area.

BRS and BRS After Dark	800-345-4277
BRS/Saunders Colleague	800-468-0908
Dialog and Knowledge Index	800-334-2564
MEDIS: Mead Data Central	800-543-6862
MEDLINE: National Library of Medicine	800-638-8480
PaperChase: Beth Isreal Hospital	800-722-2075
Grateful Med: National Technical Information Service	800-638-8480
Sci-Mate: Institute for Scientific Information	800-523-4092
SearchMaster	800-421-7229

Suggested Readings

Cox, Kenneth R. *Planning Clinical Experiments.* Springfield: Charles C. Thomas Publisher, 1968.

Drew, Clifford J. *Introduction to Designing and Conducting Research.* St. Louis: C. V. Mosby, 1980.

Goldstein, Gerald. *A Clinician's Guide to Research Design.* Chicago: Nelson-Hall Publishers, 1980.

"How to keep up with the Medical Literature: V. Access by Personal Computer to the Medical Literature." *Annals of Internal Medicine* 1505, 1986:810–24.

Isaac, Stephen, and Michael, William B. *Handbook in Research and Evaluation.* San Diego: EdITS Publishers, 1971.

Marks, Ronald G. *Designing a Research Project.* Belmont, California: Lifetime Learning Publications, 1982.

Swinscow, T. D. V. "*Statistics at Square One.*" *British Medical Journal* 1978.

3

Selection of Study Subjects

NEAL KAUFMAN

> There are more men ennobled by study than by nature.
>
> CICERO

Clinical research projects usually involve a portion (sample) of an entire group (population), and generalizations are made from this sample to describe characteristics of the whole populations. A major question facing any investigator is how to select the study subjects so that generalizations from that sample accurately reflect the whole population. This selection addresses this central issue by describing methods of sample selection and ways to estimate appropriate sample size.

Sample Selections

The choice of sampling procedures determines, in part, the validity, reliability, and generalizability of the research results (explained in detail in Chapter 5). The basic distinction is between *probability* sampling and *nonprobability* sampling. In general, samples that are selected using probability sampling more accurately reflect the total study population than samples derived using nonprobability sampling techniques.

Probability sampling assures that each subject in the population has a known chance of being included in the sample, which makes it possible for investigators to detect differences between groups of a prespecified magnitude and to estimate the probability that these differences are actually present in the study groups. It also permits accurate estimation of the sample size needed to achieve a particular degree of certainty that sample findings reflect the population from which the sample was taken.

In nonprobability sampling, there is no way to assure that each subject has a known probability of being included in the sample and no assurance that every subject has some chance of being included; therefore, the study sample may not accurately reflect the whole population. Research conclusions based on nonprobability sampling are less reliable, valid, and generalizable than those based on probability sampling. The major advantages of nonprobability sampling are convenience and low cost; advantages that might outweigh the statistical risks involved in not using probability sampling.

Regardless of which sampling technique is used, it is essential for the investigator to understand the benefits and liabilities of the selected method, to use a statistical approach appropriate for the sampling technique, and to make clearly stated definitions of which subjects are to be included in the study.

Probability Sample Techniques

Simple Random Sampling

Simple random sampling is the basic probability sampling technique, and it is incorporated into all of the more complex probability sampling designs. A simple random sample gives each element in a population an equal chance of being included in the sample and makes the selection of every possible combination of the desired number of subjects equally likely. Sample subjects are selected by using techniques such as flips of a coin, rolls of dice, or use of a table of random numbers prepared especially for this purpose. For example, assume that a hospital had 5,000 deliveries over the preceeding year and an investigator wants to obtain a 10 percent random sample of all deliveries. Each of the 5,000 cases can be assigned a unique number and then the table of random numbers marked at some random starting point (i.e., with a blind pencil stab at the page). The cases whose numbers come up as one moves from this point down the column of numbers are taken into the sample until 500 cases are selected. Random number tables can be found in almost any book on statistics.

Systematic Sampling

Systematic sampling is one simple method to obtain a random sample. After each subject is assigned a consecutive number, the investigator selects every *n*th case. This technique ordinarily works quite well, but if the subjects were not assigned the numbers randomly, the sample would also not be random. For example, if every tenth household were chosen for an interview study, the sample might not be truly random if each block were 10 houses long so that the bigger and more expensive corner houses would be selected preferentially.

Stratified Random Sampling

A stratified random sample is one in which simple random sample are selected within subcategories of a population; for example, simple random samples can be taken separately from men and from women in a large population. The main reason for choosing this type of sampling plan is the suspicion that the subcategories differ substantially on the variable of interest. Stratified random samples can be either proportionate or disproportionate, depending on whether cases are drawn in proportion to their distribution in the population. The purpose of disproportionate sampling is to make certain that there are enough cases from each group for the analysis. For example, suppose the investigator wished to study the frequency and type of seizure disorders in children who were born with low birthweight. These infants comprise a smaller proportion of the general population than normal birthweight infants. A disproportionate stratified random sample might be obtained by stratifying the population by birthweight and then randomly selecting for analyses more subjects with low birthweight. Since a specific number of low birthweight subjects would be necessary to determine the frequency of seizures disorders, this procedure would lessen the total subjects needed for the study.

Cluster Sampling

Cluster sampling is a technique that randomly samples aggregates of subjects rather than individual subjects. It is used when it is difficult or expensive to obtain a complete list of all cases. Assume, for example, that a poorly funded investigator wants to study the knowledge and attitudes of all fourth graders in a particular geographic region. The investigator might be unable to generate a comprehensive list of all fourth graders from which to randomly select the study population; however, it might be very costly to study these children because they would be scattered across many different schools. Therefore, the investigator might prepare a list of school districts stratified by size and then select a 10 percent random sample of these districts (see Figure 3.1). The schools within these districts might be stratified by ethnic breakdown and a random sample from each stratum taken. Random samples of the fourth graders within these schools would complete the process. The dangers of this type of sampling are that the investigator might stratify the sample on the wrong variables, leading to misleading conclusions.

Nonprobability Sample Techniques

Convenience Sampling

Convenience (accidental) sampling studies obtain the most readily available subjects without regard to random selection or potential bias inherent in the selection process. For example, an investigator might study all diabetic patients being seen in his or her practice. With convenience samples it is impossible to determine the probability that findings for the sample are similar to what exists in the larger population. If convenience sampling is used, one can only hope that the results are not misleading. Convenience samples are useful primarily for pilot studies or exploratory research.

Six Steps for Cluster Sampling

	<10,000 students (500 districts)			10,000–50,000 students (150 districts)			>50,000 students (60 districts)		
Stratify districts by size									
10% stratified random sample of districts	50 districts			15 districts			6 districts		
Stratify by % black population in district	20 schools (<10%)	25 schools (10–50%)	5 schools (>50%)	7 schools (<10%)	6 schools (10–50%)	2 schools (>50%)	2 schools (<10%)	2 schools (10–50%)	2 schools (>50%)
10% random sample of schools	2 schools	2 schools	1 school	1 school	1 school	1 school	1 school	1 school	1 school
Identify all 4th graders in selected schools	200 students	200 students	100 students	150 students	150 students	150 students	200 students	200 students	200 students
10% random sample of identified 4th graders	20	20	10	15	15	15	20	20	20

FIGURE 3.1. Cluster Sampling: Hypothetical Example

Quota Sampling

Quota sampling, sometimes misleadingly referred to as "representative sampling," is a type of convenience sample. It is analogous to stratified, random sampling in that a number of cases are selected from preselected strata. The selection process is, however, nonrandom and by convenience. Quota samples suffer from the same problems as other convenience samples.

Purposive Sampling

Purposive sampling involves the assumption that representative subjects can be selected by using good judgment and appropriate strategies. A common strategy is to choose cases that are judged to be typical of the population in question, assuming errors in judgment will tend to counterbalance each other; however, with no objective basis for making the judgment, this usually is not a dependable assumption.

Special Applications of Nonprobability Sampling

Given the practical realities of clinical research, nonprobability sampling will be the method used in many circumstances. While investigators recognize the superiority of random selection, many are convinced that nonprobability sampling works reasonably well despite the fact that it does not provide any basis for estimating how far the sample results deviate from true population figures.

There are circumstances in which probability sampling is unnecessary. Many samples are designed to explore ideas and gain insights rather than to determine population characteristics. Other studies seek information about motives, attitudes, and beliefs. While it might be preferable to document the distribution of these ideas in the entire population, it may not be practical or cost effective to perform such a study.

Nonprobability sampling may be chosen as a compromise with other important research considerations. For example, a better sampling method might preclude the use of a more sensitive data collection instrument. If the instrument can only be used with a person once the interviewer has become well known and accepted by the participant, it might be impractical to use random selection of participants.

Whenever nonprobability samples are used, it is critical not to use statistical procedures appropriate only for probability samples. Chapter 5 explains which methods should be used with different sampling techniques.

Combinations of Probability and Nonprobability Samples

If sampling is carried out in stages, it is possible to combine probability and nonprobability sampling in one design. An investigator may take a probability sample of subjects from a sample obtained using nonprobability techniques. For example, a number of counties may be selected for evaluation using purposive sampling and then subjects in each county selected randomly. Alternatively, an investigator may randomly select counties for evaluation and then sample cases from each county with quota sampling. Adding any randomness to the selection process will improve the degree of generalizability of the conclusions.

Sample Size

The size of the sample for a study should be large enough to show clinically relevant differences between study groups with statistical significance, and small enough to be practical and feasible. The curve shown in Figure 3.2 demonstrates the relationship between sample size and the statistical accuracy (or error) of the results. As the size of the sample increases the amount of error decreases, up to a point.

If random sampling is used, calculations can be made that estimate the sample size needed to show a particular difference between study groups at a specific degree of certainty. In order to determine sample size an investigator must be able to estimate baseline and outcome percentages (in an intervention study) or study versus control group percentages (in a comparative study) prior to starting the study. Previous studies, questionnaires, or other sources of

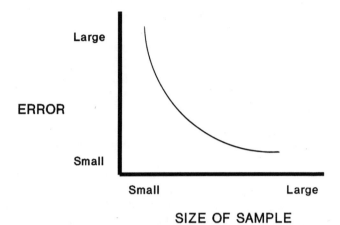

SIZE OF SAMPLE

FIGURE 3.2. Relationship between sample size and the statistical accuracy (error) of the results.

SOURCE: F. N. Kerlinger, *Foundation of Behavioral Research* (New York: Holt, Rinehart and Winston, 1973).

"educated guesses" can be used. Table 3.1 provides estimates for some sample sizes using $p < .05$ (see Chapter 5) as the level of significance value. *Baseline percentage* is the proportion of the sample with the characteristic behavior or test score present before the study or in the comparison group, and *outcome percentage* is the value after the study is completed or in the study group. *Power* refers to the probability that such a difference would be detected. That is, the power represents the likelihood that the difference between the baseline and the outcome percentage will be shown in the study samples. A power of 80 percent (.8) is usually a reasonable goal. Depending on the study, however, the researcher might increase or decrease the power. More details about power can be found in Chapter 5. Table 3.1 provides estimates for sample sizes given a baseline percentage of 10 or 50 percent for various outcome percentages and powers (assuming $p < .05$). Tables for calculating sample sizes can be found in the various texts in the Suggested Readings section of this chapter. For example, assume that 10 percent of the study population uses car seats prior to a proposed intervention. If the investigator estimates that post intervention the

TABLE 3.1. Estimated Sample Sizes for a Variable With 10 and 50%
Baseline Amounts (for Selected Outcome Percentages and Powers)

	Baseline (10%)			
%	.9	.8	.7	Power
20	236	176	139	
Outcome 25	121	91	73	
30	76	58	47	

	Baseline (50%)			
%	.9	.8	.7	Power
60	442	325	252	
Outcome 70	121	83	66	
75	70	58	42	
80	48	37	29	

Apha 0.10; two-tailed test.
Source: J. Fleiss, *Statistical Methods for Rates and Proportions* (New York: John Wiley and Sons, 1980).

value might increase to 30 percent usage and random sampling is used, then 58 subjects completing the study would give enough statistical power (.80 in this case) to state that there is an effect of the intervention. If the increased usage rate was expected to be 20 percent, the final sample size would have to be 176. These numbers should be used as estimates to help investigators determine final sample sizes before an intervention is begun. The investigator must add to these estimates the number of subjects projected not to complete the study (i.e., the attrition rate).

Sample sizes can also be calculated to show confidence intervals for samples with different percentages for particular characteristics under study. Confidence intervals give the range above and below the observed result that corresponds to specific likelihood that the answer is correct. Using confidence intervals (as opposed to *p* values only) allows the investigator not only to reject or accept a hypothesis within a known degree of uncertainty, but also to estimate the size of the treatment effect together with some measure of the uncertainty in the estimate. This helps to quantify the clinical or scientific importance of statistically significant finding by demon-

TABLE 3.2.   Confidence Intervals for Samples With Different Percentages
of a Study Characteristic and Differing Sample Sizes*

		Sample Size					
		25	50	100	200	400	800
	5	± 8	± 6	± 4	± 3	± 2	2
Sample	10	± 12	± 8	± 6	± 4	± 3	2
Percentages	20	± 16	± 11	± 8	± 6	± 4	3
	40	± 19	± 14	± 10	± 7	± 5	3

*Assumes a simple random sample, a large population, and being correct in 95 of 100 samples.
Source: K. E. Bauman, *Research Methods for Community Health and Welfare* (New York: Oxford University Press, 1980).

strating the magnitude of the difference. More details about confidence intervals can be found in Chapter 6.

Table 3.2 shows the confidence intervals obtained for different random sample sizes and differing percentages of the sample that have the characteristic under study. (This assumes that the likelihood that an answer is correct to be 95 of 100). For example, assume 20 percent of the sample have the characteristic under study and the sample size is 100. A researcher would be able to state with 95 percent confidence that the actual proportion of the total population possessing the characteristic is between 12 and 28 percent (20 ± 8 percent). The selection of what confidence level is appropriate for any particular study is problematic. Ninety-five of 100 is a typical choice. For some problems it might be necessary to increase or decrease that chance. Considerations such as cost, importance of results, and potential for inaccurate results leading to dangerous or expensive conclusions, influence the choice of the most appropriate confidence level.

Attrition of Study Subjects

In most prospective studies a number of subjects will not complete the study or will have incomplete data available. High attrition rates damage the credibility of any study and every effort should be made not to lose study subjects. Attrition rates greater than 30 percent make interpretation of the results very difficult. Generally, no attempt to replace these subjects should be made because even random selection of new subjects will not reverse potential bias caused by differential nonparticipation by study subjects. Since attrition will decrease the final sample size, the original estimate of adequate sample size must take this into account.

In order to test for bias, the investigator should compare important demographic and all known and hypothesized relevant characteristics of the individuals included and omitted from the study. Since the investigator can never be sure that all important characteristics have been evaluated, finding equivalent characteristics between the two groups may be comforting; however, it does not completely assure that bias has been eliminated. Many authors include in their paper a table showing the comparability characteristics of the two groups to lend credibility to their conclusions.

Comparative Studies: Methods for Assignment of Participants to Each Group

Comparative studies (case–controls) attempt to show that a difference in outcomes between two groups is secondary only to the intervention being studied. A proper comparison requires that the performance of the comparison group is an adequate proxy for the performance of the treatment group if they had not received the intervention. One approach to obtaining such a standard is to choose study groups that are equal or comparable with respect to all important factors except for the specific treatment.

Random Allocation

The preferred method of subject selection is random allocation. Random allocation of study subjects into comparison groups creates *control* and *experimental* groups presumed to be equivalent. Random allocation allows us to assume, within calculable limits of probability, that the groups are the same with respect to (1) the dependent variable before the independent variable was introduced and (2) variables other than those considered to be independent and dependent throughout the life of the study.

Random allocation attempts to eliminate selection bias and helps to ensure that outside influence and differences of experiences between subjects are equally distributed between experimental and control subjects. In addition, it helps to equalize maturation (natural changes in characteristics) across groups, and if regression toward the mean occurs it does so equally in experimental and control groups. It is also reasonable to assume that any influence of instrumentation or testing would be equal in each group.

For these and other reasons, random assignment is the method of choice for creation of study groups. In many circumstances, however, random assignment of subjects is not possible. In such instances matching of cases prior to the intervention can be used to help achieve equivalence of variables in which the groups differ and which are related to the dependent variable.

Matching

Matching attempts to achieve comparability because it is seldom possible to achieve equality between two matched study groups. The degree to which two groups can be made comparable depends on the difference of the distribution of the confounding variables in each group and the size of the comparison population from which one samples. The two basic approaches to forming matched groups are *pair* and *nonpair matching*. In *pair matching* a specific match (comparison subject) is found for each intervention subject. For example, each intervention subject would be matched with another subject of similar ethnicity and socioeconomic status; this subject, who does not receive treatment, is the control.

In *nonpair matching*, no attempt is made to find specific comparison subjects for each intervention subject. Two nonpair matching methods can be used: *frequency matching* and *mean matching*. In *frequency matching*, the distribution of the confounding variable in the experimental intervention group is stratified, and one attempts to equalize the number of experimental intervention and comparison subjects in each stratum. For example, assume the investigator wanted to study the effectiveness of biofeedback on the control of hypertension. If the patient's weight is hypothesized to be a confounding variable, the investigator might stratify the study group by weight and then equalize the number of study subjects in each group.

In *mean matching*, attempts are made to match the sample means for the confounding variable in question. Suppose the mean of the confounding variable in the intervention/experimental group is calculated. Control subjects would be selected to arrive at a control group whose mean score equals that of the experimental group on the confounding variable.

Once the appropriate number and types of subjects have been selected, the investigator is ready for the next step in research design (i.e., selecting the type of research model to be used).

Suggested Readings

Abramson, J. H. *Survey Methods in Community Medicine.* London: Livingston Churchill, 1974.

Anderson, S.; Auquier, A.; Hauck, W.; Oakes, D.; Vandaele, W.; and Wersberg, H. *Statistical Methods for Comparative Studies.* New York: John Wiley and Sons, 1980.

Bauman, K. E. *Research Methods for Community Health and Welfare.* New York: Oxford University Press, 1980.

Fleiss, J. *Statistical Methods for Rates and Proportions.* New York: John Wiley and Sons, 1980.

Kerlinger, F. N. *Foundations of Behavioral Research.* New York: Holt, Rinehart and Winston, 1973.

Levy, P. S., and Lemeshow, S. *Sampling For Health Professionals.* Belmont, California: Lifetime Learning Publications, 1980.

Morton, R. F., and Hebel, J. R. *A Study Guide to Epidemiology and Biostatistics.* Baltimore: University Park Press, 1984.

4

Types of Research Models and Methods

LAWRENCE WISSOW AND
JOHN PASCOE

Classifications of Study Design

Many ways have been proposed to classify and describe research study designs. Unfortunately, no one classification is entirely satisfactory and some use differing nomenclature, making it difficult for the investigator to choose from each classification what is most useful. The discussion that follows uses a traditional catalog of study designs as they are given in many standard textbooks of epidemiology. Studies are categorized by the way in which their subjects have been gathered and compared; they include the case series design, the case–control study, and the clinical trial (see Table 4.1).

In clinical research, however, few studies will fit neatly into any one of these categories. Bits and pieces of each may be used to answer a particular question. In fact; the "rules" provided for designing a particular type of study apply very broadly to nearly any design. Accordingly, two guides are provided here:

First, the list of study attributes or characteristics outlined in Table 4.2 can be used to help classify studies along several axes. In analyzing or planning a study, it is more important to consider how these attributes may apply to the question at hand than to focus on a particular study design. Second, the reader may wish to skim descriptions of all of the study designs to better understand the many points they have in common. In particular, nearly all studies require:

1. Firmly establishing a study objective or hypothesis (Chapter 2).
2. Methods of assembling groups of study subjects, including developing specific case definitions and avoiding systematic errors (bias) in the selection of study subjects (Chapter 3).
3. Making valid and reliable observations, including the consideration of biased surveillance, blinding, and variability among observers (Chapter 3).
4. Handling incomplete observations, such as individuals who are lost to follow-up, who fail to return questionnaires, or who appear to change their status (from "control" to "case," for example) during the study (Chapter 5).
5. Selecting appropriate comparison groups, including identifying and controlling for important factors that may impact on the study hypothesis (Chapter 3).

Choosing a Study Design

One of the most basic and yet difficult tasks for researchers is choosing a study design that best fits their research goals and is compatible with the methodologic resources available (time, clinical population, ethical considerations). One cannot overemphasize the importance of this task. Investigators sometimes begin a project hastily in the belief that statistical adjustments and other techniques for sifting the data can compensate for not having a very firm idea of what question is to be answered and how it is to be approached. While no study ever works as planned, and statistical techniques can compensate for unexpected trends in the results, adjustments cannot be made using data that was not collected or comparison groups that did not exist. Time spent designing a study is more than rewarded once the study is underway.

TABLE 4.1. Selected Study Designs

Case Series Design

Study Population of Cases → Study Sample of Cases → Measurement of risk factor → Level/Probability of risk factor in cases

Case–Control Study

Study Population → Study Sample(s)

↗ Cases (Have outcome of interest) → Observed Assignment → Measurement of risk factor → Level/Probability of risk factor in Cases vs. Controls

↘ Control Group(s) (Does not have outcome of interest) → Measurement of risk factor ↗

Retrospective Case–Control Study

The risk factors being compared were present in the cases and controls in the past

Cohort Study (Prospective Study)

Cross-sectional Study

The risk factors being compared are present at the time of the study

Study Population → Study Sample(s) ↗ Study Group (Exposed to Risk Factor) → Observed Assignment → Measurement of Outcome (e.g., morbidity, mortality) → Level/Probability of Outcome in the Study Group vs the Control Group

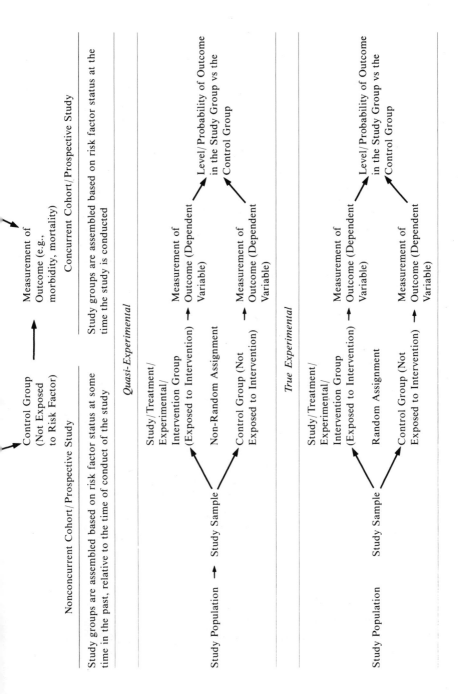

Control Group
(Not Exposed
to Risk Factor)

Measurement of
Outcome (e.g.,
morbidity, mortality)

Nonconcurrent Cohort/Prospective Study

Concurrent Cohort/Prospective Study

Study groups are assembled based on risk factor status at some
time in the past, relative to the time of conduct of the study

Study groups are assembled based on risk factor status at the
time the study is conducted

Quasi-Experimental

Study Population → Study Sample

Study/Treatment/
Experimental/
Intervention Group
(Exposed to Intervention)

Non-Random Assignment

Control Group (Not
Exposed to Intervention)

Measurement of
Outcome (Dependent
Variable)

Measurement of
Outcome (Dependent
Variable)

Level/Probability of Outcome
in the Study Group vs the
Control Group

True Experimental

Study Population   Study Sample

Study/Treatment/
Experimental/
Intervention Group
(Exposed to Intervention)

Random Assignment

Control Group (Not
Exposed to Intervention)

Measurement of
Outcome (Dependent
Variable)

Measurement of
Outcome (Dependent
Variable)

Level/Probability of Outcome
in the Study Group vs the
Control Group

41

TABLE 4.2.   Attributes of Studies

1. Strength of causation (speculation versus assertion).
2. Orientation in time.
3. Orientation to the process: prospective versus retrospective
4. Description versus comparison
5. Observation versus experimentation.

One way of trying to choose a good study design is to compare the various prototypes on several attributes that relate both to what the design can accomplish and what resources it demands (Table 4.2). Some of these attributes and how they are embodied in the basic set of clinical study designs will be discussed.

Strength of Support for a Cause–Effect Relationship

The ultimate aim of most research is to explain why events happen (i.e., to describe in detail the mechanism(s) linking a cause with a subsequent event). In general, the more the researcher can control the circumstances of a study—the way in which the study intervention is applied, the influence of other factors, the measurement of the outcome in question—the stronger one can claim to have shown evidence of causation. For example, an investigator who purposefully submits subjects to a particular intervention will have better knowledge of how the intervention was applied, and thus be more certain as to its effect, than an investigator who collects subjects who appear to have undergone the intervention in the past but might have undergone it in varying circumstances. Being able to observe a temporal relationship between two phenomena, as discussed later, is also important to asserting a cause–effect relationship.

A ranking of study designs by their causal strengths is given in Table 4.3. Many other considerations beyond the design of a single study, however, ultimately contribute to establishing a cause–effect relationship (Table 4.4).

At the initial stages of clinical research in a given area, the researcher usually encounters studies that generate rather than prove hypotheses about cause and effect. The case series, cross-

TABLE 4.3.   The Continuum of Study Designs and
Their Causal Implications

Study Designation	(1)	(2)	(3)	(4)	(5)	(6)	(7)*	Inference
Anecdotes	X			X				Speculative
Clinical hunches	X			X				
Case history	X			X				
Time series	X			X		X	X	Suggestive
Ecologic correlations	X			X		X	X	
Cross-sectional	X			X		X	X	
Case–control	X			X	X		X	Moderately suggestive
Before/after with controls	X	X			X		X	Highly
Historical cohort	X	X			X		X	suggestive
Prospective cohort	X	X			X		X	Moderately firm
Clinical randomized trials			X		X		X	Firm
Community randomized trials			X		X		X	

*(1) Observational; (2) Quasiexperimental; (3) Experimental; (4) Hypothesis generation; (5) Hypothesis testing; (6) Planning; (7) Evaluation.
Source: M. A. Ibrahim, *Epidemiology and Health Policy* (Rockville, MD: Aspen Systems Corporation, 1985), p. 40.

sectional studies, and ecologic correlations (all discussed later) are frequently used to demonstrate possible associations. Methodical reviews of previous research, known as *meta-analysis*, also can be used to generate specific hypotheses or to propose previously untested relationships. At later stages other designs such as case–control or cohort studies, which allow more precise definition of temporal relationships or individual patient characteristics, can be used to test the proposed association under more rigorous conditions.

Orientation of the Study in Time

ONE POINT IN TIME VERSUS TWO OR MORE

Most cause and effect research involves the study of phenomena that evolve over time (i.e., an agent or a process begins and subsequently an outcome or event occurs). At the early stages of a

TABLE 4.4.   Applying the Diagnostic Tests for Causation*

1. Is there evidence from true experiments in humans?

2. Is the association strong?

3. Is the association consistent from study to study?

4. Is the temporal relationship correct?

5. Is there a dose-response gradient?

6. Does the association make epidemiologic sense?

7. Does the association make biologic sense?

8. Is the association specific?

9. Is the association analogous to a previously proven causal association?

*These diagnostic tests are listed in decreasing order of their importance.
Source: D. L. Sackett, R. B. Haynes, and P. Tugwell, Clinical Epidemiology; A Basic Science for Clinical Medicine (Boston: Little, Brown and Co., 1985), p. 298.

particular line of research, the investigator may be content to observe a process at only a single point in time (Figure 4.1). Borrowing a term from anatomy, such a single-point study is often called "cross-sectional" because it can be imagined to cut across a process as that process goes on in time. It can show that two or more factors exist simultaneously in time, but the investigator can only hypothesize which came first. Observing processes at two or more points allows the investigator to better determine the sequence of events.

CONCURRENT VERSUS NONCONCURRENT

Events taking place over time can be observed from several vantage points (as shown in Figure 4.2). The standard approach is to move along in time with the process that is being observed. The intervention occurs and the researcher waits, along with the study subjects, for the outcome to take place. This orientation to time is often called *concurrent* (i.e., the researcher moves along in time in parallel with the process being observed).

Other vantage points can be taken, however. It may be that the researcher knows that an intervention or exposure has been applied in the past, and that the results are observable now, in the present. It is as if the process has gone on without the researcher, or *nonconcurrently*. The advantage of this point of view to the re-

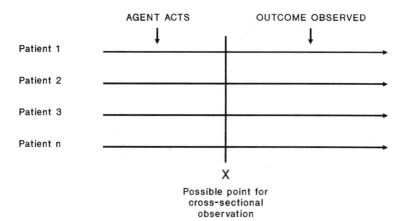

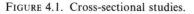

FIGURE 4.1. Cross-sectional studies.

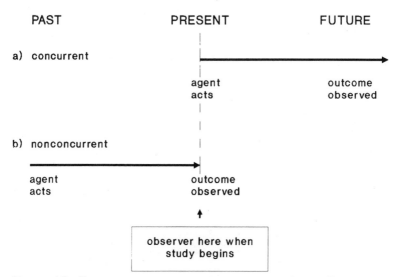

FIGURE 4.2. Concurrent versus nonconcurrent prospective studies.

45

searcher, of course, is that a question can be posed now, in the present, and not have to wait for some future outcome to be answered.

Orientation to the Process: Propsective versus Retrospective

These may be two of the most confusing terms in all of clinical epidemiology. It would seem that they relate to questions of time, as they do in everyday speech, but in fact they relate to the way in which subjects are selected for a study (Figure 4.3). In a *prospective* study, concurrent or nonconcurrent, the researcher assembles a group of individuals who will be exposed to a risk factor or intervention and then waits to observe an outcome. The majority of study designs discussed later are variations on this prospective theme. In the *retrospective* study, in contrast, the researcher selects a group of individuals expressly because they have already expe-

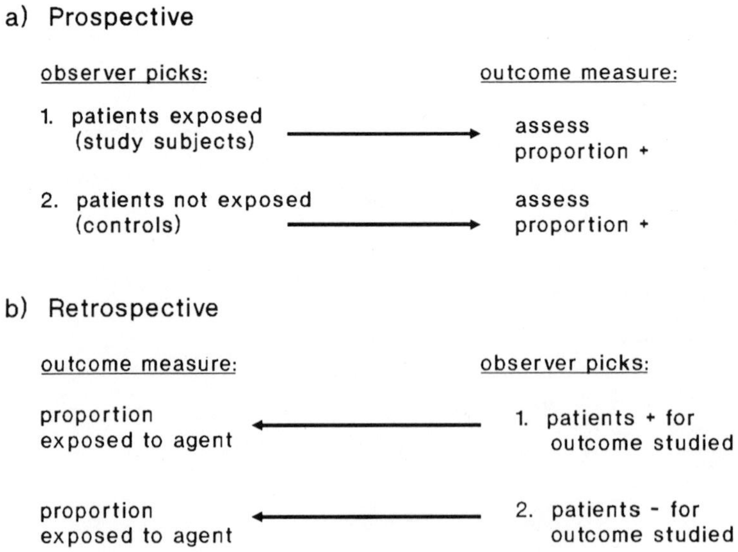

a) Prospective

observer picks: outcome measure:

1. patients exposed   ⟶   assess
   (study subjects)   proportion +

2. patients not exposed   assess
   (controls)   ⟶   proportion +

b) Retrospective

outcome measure: observer picks:

proportion   ⟵   1. patients + for
exposed to agent   outcome studied

proportion   ⟵   2. patients − for
exposed to agent   outcome studied

FIGURE 4.3. Prospective versus retrospective studies.

rienced the outcome under study. It is then asked, in retrospect, if any of them have experienced certain events that may have lead to the outcome. The case–control study is the most commonly encountered form of retrospective research. It is discussed in more detail later.

Another way to state the difference between prospective and retrospective studies is that they differ on both their orientation to time *and* what observation the investigator is trying to make. In the prospective study the researcher starts with the intervention and "waits" to observe the outcome at a later point. In a retrospective study, the researcher starts with the outcome and "looks back" to observe certain antecedent characteristics (an "intervention" or risk factor) among those experiencing the outcome.

Descriptive versus Comparative Studies

A better statement of this dichotomy is perhaps "description" versus "hypothesis testing". Descriptive studies serve to document facts that may be of clinical or theoretical significance. For example, a study describing the child-care resources available to inner city parents may be important to determine resource allocation for a health department; a study describing the natural history of otitis media may lead to hypotheses about the prevention of hearing loss. Comparative studies, on the other hand, draw contrasts between two or more groups with the intent that the comparsion will test a particular hypothesis. Mothers with better child-care resources may be postulated to have a lower failure rate for clinic appointments; it might be assumed that children with hearing loss will report having more cases of otitis than those with normal hearing.

Making comparisons is especially important in studies of clinical interventions. There are many pitfalls to simply describing the course of a group receiving treatment. Most diseases have an unpredictable outcome, and some resolve spontaneously. Subjects receiving a new treatment may respond more to the attention they receive (the "Hawthorne" and "placebo" effects) than the intervention itself. Subjects chosen because of their extreme test scores or laboratory values may appear to get better (or worse) simply because of the statistical phenomenon known as *regression to the mean*. All of these problems can be addressed by using comparative studies.

Unfortunately for a discussion of nomenclature, comparisons can be made in a descriptive way (the researcher states that the difference exists but has not generated the data in order to test any particular hypothesis), and descriptions can be used as tests of hypotheses (the researcher finds something that a hypothesis has predicted, or makes a comparison with another data set—the census, for example—that he or she did not collect). The nomenclature is imperfect but the concept is useful as a way of classifying studies. What is important is that both kinds of studies can have important scientific value when used to address the appropriate question.

Observational versus Experimental Studies

The goal of most comparative, hypothesis-testing research is to study the impact of a particular intervention or agent. In general, the researcher wants to compare the outcome when the intervention has taken place with the outcome when the intervention is absent. The intervention can occur in two ways. In one, the researcher might find naturally occurring situations in which the intervention has been differentially applied to the members of a population. For example, children living close to a smelter have received higher doses of airborne lead than have children living farther away, or children over a particular 5-year period may have received a different type of vaccine than did children immunized 5 years later. Studies involving particular outcomes in such populations are often called *observational* because they simply document processes that would be taking place without the researcher's intervention.

A second way of studying an intervention is to purposefully manipulate events. In such experimental studies, interventions are deliberately applied, and other circumstances may be altered in such a manner as to clarify the impact of the intervention. For studies to qualify as experimental, the researcher must be able to manipulate the number and range of interventions applied, at least some of the other major factors felt to influence the intervention's outcome, and the allocation of the intervention to individual study subjects. The ultimate clinical experiment, described in more detail later, is the randomized clinical trial.

In between purely observational studies and clinical trials are a number of so-called quasi-experimental methods for use when some experimental manipulations are possible, but others are not. For example, the researcher may wish to test the effectiveness of a new patient education program but cannot randomize individual patients within any given practice. The researcher can, however, choose at random which practices will test the new program and which will serve as controls. Quasi-experimental methods address the problem of how to know that any subsequently observed difference in outcome is in fact attributable to the new program and not to some inherent but unknown difference among the practices.

Descriptive Studies

The purpose of a descriptive study is to note, in greater or lesser detail, the characteristics of a group of individuals. The group may be large or small and the characteristics may pertain to the past or present. The essential feature of a descriptive study is that it does not formally test any causal hypothesis about the observed group or any comparisons that it makes with other groups. As mentioned earlier, however, descriptive studies can be used to support a hypothesis by demonstrating phenomena that the hypothesis predicts.

At their simplest, descriptive studies may involve a single patient or event—the "case report." A "case series" may describe a small group of patients thought to share one or more important attributes, such as a group having an uncommon side effect of a particular treatment. Some descriptive studies may look at the individual and aggregate characteristics of very large groups. A census, for example, is a descriptive study that has the additional aim of trying to identify and aggregate characteristics of every member of an entire population.

Descriptive studies provide much of the information on which more complex study designs rely. In fact, as Feinstein (1985) points out, the process of description is involved in all studies; other methods simply compare the descriptions of multiple groups or of the same group at multiple points in time. Feinstein lists three goals for descriptive analysis. We want to know: (1) what characteristics are present in members of the group; (2) how these characteristics are distributed among the members; and (3) how we can express these characteristics in a summary that aids comprehension and allows for later comparisons. These goals are served by keeping in mind the following requirements. They pertain as well to the observational or data-gathering steps of more complex study designs (Table 4.5).

Criteria for Inclusion in the Observed Group

Because the purpose of descriptive studies is to communicate observations about a particular population, knowing how that population was defined is essential to any subsequent interpretation of the description. Many populations in descriptive studies are simply the group of patients at a given institution who happened to receive a particular disease label. Often this process fails to include potentially eligible patients or includes those who do not deserve the label. Precise and replicable case criteria need to be established before the population is assembled.

Systematic Search of the Available Universe for Eligible Subjects

The ideal descriptive study is population based; that is, it searches every known individual in the general population for characteristics that would make him or her eligible to be in the study group. Clinical researchers may have access to such data when they use census, case registry, or other large-scale survey data, or when they attempt to pool cases of patients with certain easily diagnosable diseases from a number of neighboring institutions. In smaller settings the important tasks are first to establish case criteria and then to search the universe of available patients for those who fit the criteria.

TABLE 4.5.   General Requirements for Subject Selection
and Observation

---

1. Criteria for inclusion in the observational group must be developed.

2. A systematic search of the available universe of subjects must be made to find all those that are eligible.

3. Elements of bias in the available universe of study subjects must be assessed.

4. Rules for classifying observations must be developed and consistently applied.

Assessment of Bias in the Available Universe of Patients

Even if all the potentially eligible subjects in any particular "universe" are enumerated, the possibility exists that the group identified differs in important ways from other such groups that might be assembled in other universes; for example, it may be different in age or sex composition, or in stage of disease. Although this risk is greatest for groups assembled from a single clinic or institution, it can occur even in large-scale population-based studies. Systematic errors that lead selected groups to differ from other possible groups are called *biases*.

Bias in the context of case–control studies will be discussed in more detail later. Perhaps the most important types of bias in descriptive studies are those relating to referral patterns and to differences between actively treated patients and those who were never diagnosed or who have recovered. Both of these may lead to the development of groups that differ in major ways from the majority of patients with the same condition. Ellenberg and Nelson (1980) provide an elegant example of these biases in descriptions of the natural history of febrile seizures. By combining the results of several studies, they show that the rate at which children are found subsequently to develop chronic seizure disorders is directly related to the source of the population studied. Children with febrile seizures seen at referral centers were much more likely to have subsequent seizures than those seen in general practice. The implication of the study was that the children seen at the referral centers were different from those who had the same diagnosis but were seen in general practice. All the children had febrile seizures, but characteristics of the children and the seizures that led them to be referred for more thorough evaluation were evidently linked to a higher risk of ultimately developing a chronic seizure disorder.

Development and Consistent Application of Rules for Classifying Observations

Once patients have been included in a group, the researcher must proceed to make observations of the characteristics to be described. Just because one is merely carrying out a descriptive study does not mean that the methods of observation need not be rigorous. Even if the observations consist of record review or notation of previously collected data, criteria for inclusion and coding should be established in advance and maintained unchanged throughout the study. Ideally, if interviewing, or interpretation of narrative material is required, a worker separate from the researcher should carry out data collection. Similarly, primary sources (such as biopsy slides, radiographs, results of pulmonary function tests, interviews, or test results) should be reassessed by impartial observers instead of relying on reports. The goal is to minimize bias by those called upon to make subjective judgments. In the case of the investigator performing an interview, there is a risk that knowledge of other aspects of the research question, or convictions about the answer to the study, will consciously or unconsciously influence how the interview information is transcribed. In the case of x-ray reports, persons originally interpreting a film may have had access to other clinical information about the patient and thus not have based their interpretation on the film alone (Sackett 1985). Issues of data reliability and validity are discussed in greater detail in Chapter 5.

These requirements lead to some practical considerations for performing a descriptive study, including ways in which a clinical environment can be structured to make studies easier to carry out. First, good record systems or patient logs are needed so that the universe of patients can be enumerated. Second, these patients must be classified in ways that are relevant to the descriptive questions being addressed. In particular, the diagnostic codes frequently used in hospital settings often poorly reflect the chief complaints and diagnoses made in ambulatory care. Special classification systems have been proposed for these settings (Steinwachs 1978; Schneeweiss 1983). Third, researchers involved in descriptive studies need collaborators capable of making independent assessments of important observations, especially those that involve subjective judgments.

Cross-Sectional and Ecologic Studies

Two types of studies, the cross-sectional and ecologic, form something of a bridge between purely descriptive studies and those that can be used, even if only in limited ways, to test hypotheses. They suggest the presence of relationships, but each has a central flaw that prevents strong assertions of cause and effect. In the case of cross-sectional studies the flaw is the lack of measurement over time, and for ecologic studies it is the uncertain relationship of individual to group characteristics. These designs, however, offer certain economies of execution that make them popular ways to take first looks at new questions.

Cross-Sectional Studies

Cross-sectional designs, sometimes also called prevalence studies, are used to document comparisons among various attributes of a group, but by definition at a single point in time. As discussed earlier, the name *cross-sectional* comes from the image of taking a slice across a stream of activity that is flowing from some point of onset toward some outcome. Within that stream one may see that factor A is at such and such a level at the same time as factor B is at another level. The cross-sectional study cannot determine whether or not a change in factor A to its observed level occurred before a change in factor B (and consequently might have caused the change in B), or if, on the other hand, factor B may have changed before A. Researchers usually perform cross-sectional studies to assert that *if* it was true that factor A came before B, then a cause–effect relationship might be present. Further studies can then be carried out to prove this point.

Cross-sectional studies are the mainstay of health policy, demographic, and clinical physiologic research. Examples include measurements of the relative proportion of children in poverty versus their race, the relationship of age to peak expiratory flow rates, or the state-by-state variation in tonsillectomy rates. Many kinds of clinical information that appear to have been gathered from longitudinal studies, such as the standard children's growth chart, are often made up of cross-sectional observations. Some of the problems of using cross-sectional data in this way will be discussed later.

There are two reasons why cross-sectional studies are widely used. First and foremost is that they avoid the difficult task of tracking individuals over long periods of time, either as part of a cohort study or in a clinical trial. Sometimes longitudinal data are very difficult or impossible to obtain; for example, one does not want to wait 18 years to establish a pediatric growth chart.

Second, a great deal of cross-sectional information is available from public sources. The Census, surveys conducted by the National Center for Health Statistics, Medicaid and insuranace company payment files, and hospital discharge data all lend themselves to cross-sectional analysis. Often this is the only kind of analysis possible because identifiers needed for longitudinal analyses are either unavailable or cannot be released for study purposes.

Three major weaknesses often limit cross-sectional studies to early stages in the exploration of hypotheses. First, if the study involves groups of persons with different ages or stages of disease, so-called cohort effects may cause the investigator to reach false conclusions. The apparently homogeneous group of individuals may in fact be made of subgroups (cohorts) who were subjected to differing risks or who have been given differing treatments. To use Lilienfeld's example (1980, pp. 118–20), a general population cross-sectional study of tuberculin skin-test reactions versus age may find that older individuals more frequently have positive tests, suggesting that the risk of tuberculosis increases sharply with old age. In fact, since one's status as a skin-test reactor lasts for life, it may be that the cohort of individuals now older than 65 years of age was exposed to tuberculosis in their youth, at a time when the disease was more widespread. Reactions among younger individuals, who grew up when the disease was less prevalent, more accurately reflect current exposure.

By far the biggest problem of cross-sectional studies is their inability to show temporal sequence in support of a claim of causality. These studies show associations, the simultaneous occurrence of two or more characteristics in an individual or group. Unfortunately, many events seem to occur simultaneously but have no fixed association with each other. Although this problem can never be overcome, careful formulation of hypotheses and alternative hypotheses plus careful planning of the study can add considerable weight to the findings. The researcher attempting to show a causal relationship must prove not only that the data support the study hypothesis but also that they do not fit (or not as well) competing alternative hypotheses. Furthermore, the researcher must show that the correlations observed also apply to other variables that seem logically related. For example, suppose that a cross-sectional study was designed to support the hypothesis that poverty is related to the severity of childhood asthma. It might initially be observed that hospitalization rates for asthma are elevated in counties with low-income populations. It would be equally important to show that the elevated rates could not be fully explained by alternative explanations, such as differences in the availability of medical services. It would also help the assertion of a relationship to show that the poorer counties with high asthma rates also had high rates of other conditions whose relationship to poverty was already somewhat established. In short, researchers performing cross-sectional studies must be careful to show that they have not simply sifted the data until they found a relationship that fit their needs.

Another problem sometimes encountered when cross-sectional studies use "found" data from public sources is that the researcher must be prepared to defend the validity of the data. This is especially true when the data are derived from billing or management information systems not originally designed for research purposes. While data specially collected for a study can often be rigidly controlled and sometimes checked against independent sources, previously acquired data sets are usually limited to internal checks on their validity. These bootstrap methods include looking for nonsense entries (such as males with hysterectomies or octagenerian preschoolers), comparing key descriptive variables with comparable populations reported in the literature, and searching for systematic changes (either at a point in time or involving a particular subset of the population) that suggest systematic errors in data collection or coding. This type of problem may be worse for particular areas of study; for example, gastroenteritis or dehydration may be less reliably coded as discharge diagnoses than the fact that a herniorraphy or appendectomy was performed.

Ecologic Studies

Sometimes, when planning a study, an investigator is unable to obtain information on a particular factor for each person participating in the study. One may wish to study the relationship between diet and heart disease, for example, but have no individual data on what people eat. It may be known, however, that persons in group A ate an average of 5 pounds of meat per month, while those in group B ate an average of 10 pounds. This type of data is known as *ecologic* because one knows about the group's environment, but not necessarily about the exposure of any individual member of the group. Investigations that use this form of data are called *ecologic studies*.

Cross-sectional studies of large population groups frequently make use of ecologic data, treating the information as if it had actually been aggregated from individual values. The study relating rates of heart disease to per capita meat consumption is a classic example. One knows that country A with a low per capita meat consumption has a low rate of heart disease, while country B with high consumption has high rates. The heart disease rates are calculated from individual mortality data, but the information on meat consumption is based on statistics of sales by slaughterhouses, divided by the population of each country. A preliminary conclusion is that consumption of meat is related to the incidence of heart disease. Such a study, however, is subject to the so-called ecologic fallacy: because we do not know about the meat consumption of individuals who did or did not die of heart disease, we cannot be certain that the association of these two factors at a national level is not caused by some third variable of which we are unaware. Of course, even if we had data on individual meat consumption we still might be left with this question, but we would be more certain that meat eating was in some way associated with heart disease on an individual basis, if only as a marker for some other truly causal factor.

Ecologic variables may be used in many study designs, not just those that are cross-sectional. They are frequently found in time-series analyses (described later along with other quasi-experimental designs). An example is the assessment of the changing impact of regional perinatal care, where the ecologic variable is the supply of perinatal services as they vary over time, perhaps measured as NICU beds per capita.

Comparative Studies

Observational

CASE–CONTROL STUDIES
Case–control studies represent the next level beyond cross-sectional designs in the attempt to show causal relationships. Case–control

studies are sometimes called *retrospective* studies because they work backwards along a potential causal chain, starting from the outcome of interest and working back toward uncovering differential rates of some exposure. In a case–control study the investigator starts with a group of individuals who already have experienced an outcome and one or more groups who have not. The investigator tries to find the proportion in each having had a certain exposure. The hypothesis of causation is supported if the proportion of subjects exposed is greater in the group with the outcome under study (the "cases") compared to the proportion among those who were selected because they had not experienced the outcome (the "controls").

A variant of the case–control study uses pairs of patients, one case associated with one or more control individuals who are "matched" to the case on several factors (such as age or sex). In this setting, the outcome is determined by the proportion of pairs for which the exposure status of the case and control are different.

There are several reasons why an investigator might want to adopt a case–control framework for research. First, when a study involves an outcome that occurs infrequently, an investigator might need to follow a very large group of at-risk subjects forward in time. Similarly, if an outcome occurs long after exposure the investigator might not be able to follow the group for a long enough period, or may feel that an answer to the research question is needed more urgently. Case–control studies address these difficulties by starting at the end of the process and identifying existing cases rather than waiting for them to happen. Case–control studies are also useful for efficiently examining multiple risk factors that could contribute to the same outcome, although care must be taken to have a large enough sample size for each of the factors to be assessed (see Chapter 3). Most of all, case–control studies are appealing for their potential economy. Usually study subjects need be contacted only once to answer questions about past exposures. In prospective studies multiple contacts and elaborate tracking systems are often needed to assess the subjects in their baseline and subsequent conditions.

Case–control studies also have some disadvantages. First, their results can only give approximations of the actual rates with which the outcome occurs. This is because the rate of a given outcome, as determined in a prospective study, is given by:

$$\frac{\text{number with the outcome}}{\text{number exposed (or "at risk")}}$$

In contrast, what a case–control study finds is:

$$\frac{\text{number with the exposure}}{\text{number of persons with the outcome}}$$

Whereas a comparative prospective study ultimately yields a measure of relative risk (see Chapter 6), the case–control study yields a measure known as *relative odds*, or the odds ratio. Both measures give an indication of the strength of the relationship between the exposure and outcome, but only under some circumstances are they numerically equivalent.

A second problem is that determining an individual's past exposure to an event or risk factor is not as reliable as making that determination in the present. Uncertainty always exists, and the investigator is never sure of how an individual came to be exposed, given the exposure is often not a random event. Additionally, persons who are "cases" may have an increased memory for certain past events that they believe are related to their condition, and thus may be more likely than control subjects to report an exposure.

A third problem is that the outcome of a case–control study is dependent on the selection of an appropriate control group. Unfortunately, it is usually not clear which control group would be the best or if the one selected was adequate. Thus case–control studies may be found less than convincing by skeptical readers.

The design of a case–control study can be seen as having five major steps: hypothesis development, establishment of definitions, case selections, control selection, and exposure determination. Although these steps are common to nearly all study designs, they have been most completely described in the context of case–control studies. More complete discussions are available in the books by Feinstein (1985, Chapter 23), Lilienfeld (1980, Chapter 8), and Sackett (1979).

OBSERVATIONAL COHORT STUDIES

As discussed previously, the often confusing terms *prospective* or *longitudinal* study are used to describe designs in which groups of patients are identified at the time of some exposure or event and then followed forward in time to determine an outcome. Also discussed previously was the idea that prospective studies could be either concurrent (that is, moving along with the researcher in real time) or nonconcurrent (constructed from exposure events in the past in order to have the outcome measureable in the present). Prospective studies may also be classified in a second way, either as observational cohort studies or as experimental clinical trials. The following paragraphs will discuss observational studies; clinical trials will be discussed later.

In a cohort study (*cohort* from the Latin for "a group of warriors"), individuals with certain baseline characteristics are observed from this baseline until a previously defined endpoint is reached. Observational cohort studies can be carried out in four general ways:

Single heterogeneous group followed from baseline to outcome. Cohorts for this type of study are usually chosen because they are homogeneous for one or more characteristics (such as date of birth, place of residence, or socioeconomic status), but heterogeneous for other characteristics that may relate to the outcome being studied (such as occupation or exposure to a drug or toxin). At the time that outcome is assessed, one hopes to find a relationship among the heterogeneous characteristics and the outcome. This type of study is *comparative* in that it contrasts outcome among subjects who do or do not possess the heterogeneous characteristics. It is *observational* in that it does not deliberately allocate the heterogeneous characteristics, such as drug exposure, as might be done in a clinical trial.

This type of design is often used in studies that wish to examine the precursors and natural history of a particular condition. For example, Altemeir and co-workers (1982) assembled a group of mothers who were all of similar socioeconomic status and who were giving birth in the same hospital. They interviewed the mothers and then followed the children as they grew up. Ultimately, some of the mothers abused or neglected their children, and the investigators were able to look at characteristics of the mothers at the time of their child's birth that were more common among those who later became abusive.

Two homogeneous groups followed from baseline to outcome. Strictly speaking, a cohort study of this design is an example of Campbell and Stanley's (1963) "nonequivalent control group" quasi-experimental design (see later). In this design, the researcher assembles a cohort of subjects who all have a condition or characteristic of interest, such as a history of failure to thrive in infancy. A control cohort is then assembled of children with normal growth in infancy, but who are otherwise similar to the other cohort in sex, maternal age, and socioeconomic status. The two cohorts are followed to a specified outcome (for example, developmental tests at entry to preschool) at which time comparisons can be made in the outcome measure.

The purely descriptive cohort study. A descriptive cohort study may follow only one group and document certain attributes as they change over time. A longitudinal study of blood pressure or linear growth in pediatric patients is one example of this type of design. If the study is purely descriptive no attempt will be made to identify patient characteristics responsible for the pattern of change over time, or to draw contrasts between subgroups who have different patterns of change.

Epidemiologic cohorts. The three kinds of cohort studies described earlier all follow the paths of individual patients and assess their status at two or more points in time. Epidemiologists, however, sometimes use the term *cohort study* to look at the aggregate characteristics of groups at two or more points in time without identifying the fate of any particular individual. For example, demographers might want to examine how the birth rate of a cohort of women who were aged 15–20 years in 1965 varies as the women grow older. Birth certificates would be examined and a rate calculated for women of this age group in 1965, for women aged 20–25 years in 1970, and so on. No individuals are identified, but it is assumed that those included in each of the successive calculations all belong to the same group.

What separates all four of the study types from clinical trials is that the agent or intervention under study has been applied by nature and not deliberately by the researcher. Thus two of the major tasks facing the researcher using an observational cohort design, in parallel to the problems encountered for case–control studies, are to be certain that no biases were operating at the time subjects were being exposed to the agent and that exposure did, in fact, take place. In spite of these difficulties, cohort studies, especially those involving a single heterogeneous group followed from baseline to outcome, have several advantages over the types of studies discussed thus far. First, given the proper selection of study groups, they allow direct calculation of incidence or morbidity rates instead of an odds ratio. Second, prospective studies allow the most unambiguous determination of temporal sequence, especially if they are performed concurrently. Third, the researcher can often design a study so that several different kinds of outcomes can be determined at the same time. For example, a longitudinal study of anxious attachment in infancy may be able to look at educational, social, and emotional outcomes all within the same cohort.

Prospective studies do have potential drawbacks. They work best when the exposure measured is relatively rare but has a high attack rate. This allows the investigator to easily find unexposed controls and have a relatively small exposed group to track. It might be difficult, for example, to perform a study to detect late and subtle pulmonary sequelae of children exposed to varicella virus. It would be hard to find controls (i.e., children never exposed to varicella), and the researcher would have to follow a large group of people because the outcomes observed are known to be rare. On the other hand, a study of the sequelae of severe head injury might be relatively easy. A large number of subjects without a history of serious injury would be available, and most of those injured would be expected to have some recognizable impairment within a relatively short period of time. Nonconcurrent prospective studies avoid some of these constraints by avoiding the problem of tracking subjects. On the other hand, they risk biases similar to those found in case–control studies when one attempts to ascertain past exposure.

Sackett and co-authors (1985, p. 161) have outlined a procedure for evaluating a published account of a prospective study. The outline can also be used as a framework for planning a study, and includes: (1) assembling the initial cohort; (2) devising a scheme for tracking the cohort's members; (3) developing objective outcome criteria; (4) developing an unbiased method of ascertaining outcome status; and (5) measurement of other factors (confounders) that might influence the outcome.

Experimental Studies

Since their "discovery" only a few decades ago, clinical trials have come to be considered the gold standard of biomedical research. The term *clinical trial* is most often used to refer to a study whose design incorporates five key elements:

1. It is a concurrent, prospective comparison of two or more groups;
2. One or more of the groups is deliberately exposed to an intervention, usually a medical therapy, while at least one group (the controls) is not exposed or receives a more standard therapy;
3. The study groups are generated from a single, homogeneous pool of subjects. Assignment of individuals to each experimental or control group is determined by a method based on random events and without any consideration of which member of the pool is assigned to which group;
4. All study participants (subjects, treating clinicians, and outcome evaluators) are unaware of which subjects are receiving an intervention and which are in a control group. This "blinding" may also extend to various participants being unaware of the true study hypothesis or the nature of the outcome measure;
5. Control subjects receive an intervention that is either indistinguishable (to the subjects) from the actual intervention or is felt to have equivalent impact in ways that might effect the outcome to be measured. This usually includes attention to psychologic factors such as the placebo or Hawthorne effects through which some outcomes or behavior may change because individuals believe that they are being treated or because they know that they are being observed. In general, control and experimental groups should both experience some form of intervention and have an equivalent amount of contact with the research staff.

Clinical trials are ideally suited to some kinds of studies, but they have limited or no usefulness for others. The setting in which they work best is in trials of therapy for subjects with known diseases, what Feinstein calls *remedial trials* (Feinstein 1983). This setting works so well because the subjects usually have in common some easily defined characteristic that would be expected to change rapidly and visibly in response to treatment. This makes it relatively easy for the investigator to find a uniform subject pool with which to begin, and to conduct the study over a manageable period of time with the smallest possible group of subjects. These considerations were discussed previously in the context of observational cohort studies.

Clinical trials are less suited to studies of preventive measures. In this type of study the time to outcome may be lengthy, and it may be impossible to keep subjects from being exposed to other treatments or activities that could have an impact on outcome. Nevertheless, clinical trials have been conducted in both cancer and cardiovascular disease prevention, to name but two examples.

Clinical trials are poorly suited to studies of: (1) multiple therapeutic modalities (because too many subjects are needed to evaluate the many possible therapeutic combinations); (2) small changes in a therapeutic plan (the effort it takes to do the study may outweigh the potential significance of the outcome); (3) therapies that may be changed during the course of the study so that the results are at risk for becoming obsolete before the study is completed; and (4) treatments with only rare outcomes or outcomes that will only be observable at a time far distant in the future. This last situation is of critical importance because it underlines the fact that clinical trials rarely produce good information about the adverse effects of therapies. It may take a clinical trial of only a few hundred patients to demonstrate the efficacy of a new antibiotic, for example, if the drug has a relatively dramatic effect on the condition it is used to treat. If the drug has a significant side effect on 1 or 2 of every 1,000 subjects treated, however, the chances of observing that side effect during the trial are small. Thus proving both the efficacy *and* safety of a new drug may take both a clinical trial (to demonstrate efficacy) and a case–control or long-term observational cohort study to find infrequent or latent side effects.

Ethical considerations may also limit the use of clinical trials. Obviously noxious exposures cannot be purposefully tested on humans, and some potentially noxious therapies may not be appropriate for trials with children or others unable to give consent themselves. Likewise, situations in which subjects are coerced to participate, even just to be in the control group, violate the patient's right to personal choice in seeking health care.

A frequently difficult area is the testing of a therapy that has already had widespread clinical use. At this point many practitioners object that it would be unethical to deprive therapy to a patient, something that could happen if the patient is assigned to a control group in a clinical trial. There are several approaches to resolving this problem. First, it is noteworthy that the accepted nature of a therapy is often a function of the clinician who uses it. Finding a way to test the therapy in someone else's domain may suffice. For example, one researcher found that a study of decongestants as therapy for the common cold could not be carried out in the offices of private practitioners because these physicians believed unequivocally that decongestants were useful. The study was carried out, however, with the approval of an institutional review board, in a teaching clinic where decongestants were not routinely prescribed.

Alternatively, the close examination of patient selection and outcome measurement methods in previous, uncontrolled trials that appear to support the therapy may show flaws that someone is willing to subject to a test. Studies can also be designed that involve carefully monitored delay in definitive treatment while an alternative is administered. Whether any of these approaches is likely to succeed is frequently dependent on the perspective of the institutional review board or clinical research committee at the facility involved.

All the aspects of designing a clinical trial suffer from one central dilemma: balancing the study's internal purity (statistical and methodologic rigor) with its external validity (the degree of generalization possible or the clinical usefulness of the results). Feinstein discusses this point in detail in his book (1985, Chapter 29) and in his series of papers in the *Annals of Internal Medicine* (1983). In general, efforts to achieve extreme methodologic purity can result in studies that are either impossible to perform or so narrowly focused that they are useless to most clinicians. On the other hand, the validity of loosely designed studies that seem to show important results may often be rightfully challenged. It is important to address this dilemma at each stage of study design. These as well as many other practical considerations are discussed at length in the book by

Meinert, *Clinical Trials* (1986). A few considerations that are unique to clinical trials include:

DEFINING THE ELIGIBLE POPULATION AND SELECTING SUBJECTS
FROM IT BEFORE EXPERIMENTAL/CONTROL STATUS IS ASSIGNED
As with all types of studies, the ability to use the findings of a clinical trial depends heavily on how the study group was assembled and what population it represents. Perhaps the most important point for clinical trials is that eligible subjects be recruited before their treatment assignment is determined. This guards against biases in recruiting and differential refusal rates for study and control subjects.

DEVELOPMENT OF THE TREATMENT PROTOCOL
The central problem in this step is to design a protocol that asks a clinically relevant question, is easily replicable, is capable of being "blinded," and is resistant to drift or change during the course of the study. Some protocols involve a single act or intervention while others may require a long course of treatment. Almost all must consider the possibility that other interventions will be required either to deal with complications of the treatment or to respond to new problems. Other treatments that are permitted, and how these treatments can be documented, must be determined prior to the start of the study.

A major problem in many drug trials, for example, is that the dose of the drug must be adjusted to optimal serum levels or to obtain a visible clinical response. Ideally, a plan must be devised that allows realistic clinical manipulation of the drug dose without giving away the fact that the patient is receiving the active agent. The extreme alternative of simply prescribing a fixed dose usually will not result in a satisfactory trial of the drug. Similar problems are involved in trials that compare invasive versus drug or behavioral therapies. Often the investigator must settle for a study that is only partially blinded but where randomization is rigorous, the subjects in the various study arms do not have a chance to observe one another, and where at least outcome assessment is blind to the intervention given.

SELECTING ALTERNATIVE TREATMENTS
The internal/external validity dilemma becomes important at this stage in the choice of comparing the experimental intervention with

a placebo (is the new therapy demonstrably different from making no intervention?) or with another active form of treatment (is the new therapy significantly different from existing care?). The former strategy often results in study outcomes of greater magnitude while the latter may provide information that is more useful clinically.

A potential variant is to use a *cross-over design* in which subjects are exposed sequentially to both the active treatment and a control or placebo intervention (Louis 1984). For example, a study of a low-dose muscle relaxant taken for headaches may involve alternating courses of a placebo and the active drug. Subjects are asked to continually rate the severity of their headaches but are not told when the treatment is being changed. This kind of structure has great appeal because the subjects can be their own control and because all subjects can potentially benefit from the intervention. Cross-over studies also have the potential to require much smaller sample sizes than conventional parallel clinical trials. Not all interventions can be tested in this manner, however. The intervention must be known not to be influenced by trends over time. Such trends may involve either the evolution of the patient's condition or outside influences (such as season on children's blood lead levels) that may effect the outcome independently of the treatment. In addition, the intervention should have no carry-over effect beyond the time it is administered. Otherwise subsequent control periods will not be truly without therapy. In practice, cross-over studies may employ a washout period between switches during which time results are not assessed, and will also randomly assign subjects to various alternations of control and treatment periods. It is also important to consider the rules governing when subjects cross to the opposite therapy. It is generally agreed that switches should take place at predetermined time intervals and not at times set by the subject's response or disease state.

QUASI-EXPERIMENTAL STUDIES

Campbell and Stanley (1963) popularized the term *quasi-experimental* for study designs that deviated from the ideal of random assignment to treatment and control groups. In the social and behavioral sciences, they noted, the intransigency of the research environment frequently did not allow the degree of manipulation required for classic experimentation. The major intransigencies they encountered (though not all at once, fortunately!) were:

1. The inability to randomize individual study subjects;
2. The availability of only a single study group;
3. The prohibition of keeping one group as a control (being required to provide all groups with some intervention); and
4. The inability of pre-testing any of the groups to determine baseline characteristics.

Campbell and Stanley did not consider these limitations to be prohibitions to meaningful research. Their approach was dictated by two major precepts. First, they reminded their readers that single studies, even using ideal experimental conditions, rarely provided all the information needed to answer a clinically meaningful question. Thus there was nothing wrong with planning a study that would not yield a "final" answer. What mattered was that the results be obtained in a defensible manner and that they be capable of being integrated into the larger body of work pertaining to the study question. It would be the trend of multiple studies that would ultimately provide any possible approximation to the truth.

Their second principle was similar to the points discussed previously pertaining to cross-sectional studies. In the absence of an explicit test for causality, the investigator could compensate by examining the internal consistency of the results and by specifically considering how the data fit with competing hypotheses. To the extent that the data failed to support alternative hypotheses, and within any obvious limits of the study's design, the conclusions should be worthy of serious consideration.

Campbell and Stanley outlined several quasi-experimental designs and rated them for resistance to a variety of threats to validity. These threats included trends in both subject response and outside influences over time, test–retest effects, regression to the mean, and selection bias.

Knowledge of the potential threats for each design is important because a specific threat usually suggests one or more alternatives to the hypothesis under consideration. If a given design will not allow testing of an alternative that seems important, another design might be selected. The reader is referred to Campbell and Stanley's text itself for a full discussion. Brief mention of some of the possible designs is made in the following paragraphs. A few of the many possible combinations of intransigency are considered and a possible study design for each is discussed. The purpose of these paragraphs is to give a flavor for the design possibilities, not to give a complete explanation of how to use them.

INTRANSIGENCY NUMBER ONE:

- Randomization of individuals is not possible but multiple groups are available.
- Pretesting is possible so that equivalency of the groups can be assessed.
- It is permissible simply to observe one of the groups and thus use it as a control.

Such a situation is frequently encountered in health services research where two or more clinic or geographically described populations must be compared, one receiving the intervention (often a new clinical service) and the other continuing with standard practices. Even though individual patients cannot be randomized, this setting allows the closest approximation to a randomized trial. Campbell and Stanley called it the *nonequivalent control group design* because the major threat to validity is that the control population risks not being equivalent, and thus comparable, to the study group. To use their notation, where "O" indicates a period of observation and "X" a period of intervention, this design would be drawn:

$$\begin{array}{c c c c}
\text{group 1} & \underline{\quad 0 \quad X \quad 0 \quad} \\
\text{group 2} & \quad 0 \quad \quad \; 0 \quad
\end{array}$$

where the line indicates that the groups are not randomized and are thus potentially nonequivalent. To the extent that the groups can be shown to be equivalent, the design does closely approach a real experiment. Most of the cautions that apply to randomized clinical trials apply to this quasi-experimental variant as well.

As a historical note, the nonequivalent control group design may be one of the oldest recorded types of human experimentation (Feinstein 1985). As Daniel told King Nebuchadnezzar's guard:

"Please test your servants for ten days, giving us legumes to eat and water to drink. Then compare our appearance with that of the youths who eat of the king's food. . . ." When the ten days were over, they looked better and healthier than all the youths who were eating of the king's food. (Daniel 1.12–16)

INTRANSIGENCY SITUATION NUMBER TWO:

- Individual randomization is not possible.
- Multiple groups are available but all must get an intervention (more than one is possible).
- Pretesting may or may not be possible.

For this situation Campbell and Stanley propose a variety of counterbalanced designs. The basic principle is that several groups are each administered several treatments, each group receiving the treatments in a different order (similar to a cross-over clinical trial). If the experiment is replicated enough times, using many of the possible combinations of ordering the treatments, it should be possible both to identify a treatment that is consistently superior and to convince oneself that the superiority is not an artifact of either ordering or time trends. A diagram of the study might look like this:

	time 1	time 2	time 3	time 4
group 1	X1 0	X2 0	X3 0	X4 0
group 2	X2 0	X3 0	X4 0	X1 0
group 3	X3 0	X4 0	X1 0	X2 0
group 4	X4 0	X1 0	X2 0	X3 0

This study would have many of the limitations discussed previously for cross-over designs. Any sort of treatment that had lasting effects, or measurement methods with significant test–retest effects, would be unsuitable. The main strength of such studies is in their demonstration of consistency. The more permuations explored in which a given treatment seems best, the harder it is to support challenges to the study's validity.

INTRANSIGENCY SITUATION NUMBER THREE:

• No randomization of individuals is possible.
• Pretesting is possible.
• There is only one group to be observed.

This situation may require the use of the time–series or equivalent time–samples designs. In the time–series design, multiple observations of a group are made over a period of time. At some point an intervention is introduced and multiple observations continue. The researcher then tries to explain changes seen after the intervention as attributable to it. The Campbell and Stanley diagram looks like this: O O O O X O O O O. The major difficulty with this method is in trying to prove that the postintervention changes would not have happened anyway. Various graphic and mathematical approaches are possible to show that the postintervention changes would not have been predicted from the preintervention trend of the observations. The researcher must also assert that no external event happened coincidentally with the intervention and was really responsible for the observed change.

The equivalent time–samples design addresses these points. It is essentially a one-armed cross-over study where the treatment group alternates two or more times from baseline to intervention and back. The diagram might be drawn: O O X O O X O O X O O. At this point if change is observed after the intervention, and especially if the observed characteristic then returns to baseline, natural trends or outside influences become much less likely explanations.

Guyatt and co-workers (1986) have recently proposed using this kind of design for the assessment of treatment effects in single patients, the so-called *n* of 1 trial. A consultation service at McMaster University has been established to allow patients to test, in a blinded fashion, their response to medications such as bronchodilators or psychotropics where it may be difficult to determine if the drug is actually useful. The patient and his or her clinician both agree to be blinded to an alternating series of drug and placebo (or alternative drugs). They also agree to a protocol for observing the patient's clinical status. At the end of the trial the consultant breaks the code and shares the results.

The term *time–series analysis* is also applied to a technique often applied to large-scale population data. In this setting, attempts are made to explain trends over time in a particular observation (such as the overall mortality rate of a population). Using data—often ecologic—on potential explanatory variables (such as the proportion of persons living in poverty or the rate of unemployment) computer routines derive mathematical formulas linking change in the variables with change in the outcome. Such analyses may be useful in suggesting further studies or in projecting future trends.

With luck the reader has not yet become discouraged trying to sort the many factors that enter into the selection of a study design for a particular question. Needless to say, the better focused the study question and the more precisely framed the hypotheses, the more likely it is that a particular design will suggest itself. The many practical and ethical considerations outlined elsewhere in this manual will also come into play.

Some examples of questions and the methods of research that might be used are shown in the following:

Question	*Method*
1. What is the history of infant feeding practices in the United States?	Descriptive Review Paper
2. What anticipatory guidance is given for injury control on routine checkups?	Case Studies
3. What is the pattern of growth in children with Down Syndrome?	Observational (longitudinal) Cohort
4. What are the characteristics of teenage youngsters on probation for drug abuse?	Cross-Sectional
5. What is the relationship of dietary counseling during well-baby checks to iron deficiency anemia in infants?	Cross-Sectional or Quasi-Experimental
6. What is the influence of policy on mean family income and hospital days per child using aggregated data?	Ecologic
7. Is prednisone combined with trimethoprim-sulfamethoxazole more effective in resolving persistent middle ear effusions than trimethoprim-sulfamethoxazole alone?	Clinical Trial
8. What is the change in injury potential in a group of infants after parents are given an educational program? (assuming some factors such as maturation, selective attrition, effects of testing, etc., are unavoidable.)	Quasi-Experimental

For most questions, the choice of design is an interative process. First, an initial design is suggested by the question and by the available research settings and resources. Then the reseacher must carefully consider the biases and limitations inherent in that design and what impact they have on the study's goals. Often a new design must be selected or the study's goal revised. Needless to say, time spent on this stage of the study is greatly rewarded both during the execution of the study and when the moment comes to analyze and interpret outcome data.

Suggested Readings

Introduction

Feinstein, A. R. *Clinical Epidemiology: The Architecture of Clinical Research*. Philadelphia: W. B. Saunders, 1985. A very useful book, although because Feinstein has developed a new vocabulary of methodologic principles it is not always easy to understand. The author is the leading proponent of the "architecture" approach to classifying research design.

Fletcher, R. H.; Fletcher, S. W.; and Wagner, E. H. *Clinical Epidemiology—The Essentials*. Baltimore: Williams and Wilkins. 1982. A popular and readable text with good, concise descriptions of various types of studies.

Light, R. J., and Pillemer, D. B. *Summing Up: The Science of Reviewing Research*. Cambridge: Harvard University Press, 1984. A readable and useful book about the art and science of writing review articles and the technique of "meta–analysis."

Lilienfeld, A. M., and Lilienfeld, D. E. *Foundations of Epidemiology*. 2nd ed. New York: Oxford University Press, 1980. One of the standard texts, dividing studies into those that are observational versus experimental and prospective versus retrospective.

Michael, M.; Boyce, W. T.; and Wilcox, A. J. *Biomedical Bestiary: An Epidemiologic Guide to Flaws and Fallacies in the Medical Literature*. Boston: Little, Brown and Co., 1984. An approachable and concise listing of some of the major pitfalls in clinical research design; a little "cutesy" at times but especially good for its concrete examples of the problems, lists of actual studies in which the problems occur, and suggested readings.

Sackett, D. L.; Haynes, R. B.; and Tugwell, P. *Clinical Epidemiology: A Basic Science for Clinical Medicine.* Boston: Little, Brown and Co., 1985. In general an excellent book for both beginners and advanced workers.

Descriptive Studies

Ellenberg, J. H., and Nelson, K. B. "Sample Selection and the Natural History of Disease: Studies of febrile seizures." *JAMA* 243 (1980):1337.

Moses, L. E. "The Series of Consecutive Cases as a Device for Assessing Outcomes of Intervention. *N Engl J Med* 311(1984):705–10. Some "rules" for writing up a case series.

Schneeweiss, R. et al. "Diagnosis Clusters: a New Tool for Analyzing the Content of Ambulatory Medical Care." *Med Care* 21(1983):105–22.

Steinwachs, D. M., and Mushlin A. I. "The Johns Hopkins Ambulatory Care Coding Scheme. *Health Serv Res* 13(1978):36–49.

Cross-Sectional Studies

Berger, L. R. "Abortions in America: The Effects of Restrictive Funding." *N Engl J Med* 298(1979):1474–77. A classic example of the powerful policy uses of cross-sectional, descriptive data.

Cohort Studies

Altemeir, W. A.; O'Connor, S.; Vietze, P. M.; Sandler, H. M.; and Sherrod, K. B. Antecedents of Child Abuse." *J Pediatr* 100(1982):823–29. An example of an observational cohort study.

McConnochie, K. M., and Roghmann, K. J. "Bronchiolitis as a Possible cause of Wheezing in Childhood: New Evidence." *Pediatrics* 74(1984):1–10. An example of a nonconcurrent or "historical" cohort study.

Case–Control Studies

Sackett, D. L. "Bias in Analytic Research." *J Chronic Dis* 32(1979):51–63. This is one of the "classics" in its enumeration of the types of bias.

Schlesselman, J. J. *Case–Control Studies: Design, Conduct, Analysis.* New York: Oxford University Press, 1982. A widely used text if you want an entire book on this kind of study. See also useful chapters in Lilienfeld, Feinstein, and review articles referenced in Michael, Boyce and Wilcox.

Clinical Trials

Armitage, P. *Sequential Clinical Trials.* New York: John Wiley and Sons, 1975. This and the following reference discuss the dilemmas of "multiple looks" at data coming from an ongoing clinical trial.

Dupont, W. D. "Sequential Stopping Rules and Sequentially Adjusted p Values: Does One Require the Other?" *Cont Clin Trials* 4(1983):3–10. Not light reading.

Feinstein, A. R. "An Additional Basic Science for Clinical Medicine; II. The Limitations of Randomized Trials." *Ann Intern Med* 99(1983):544–50. Readable and general.

Louis, T. A.; Lavoir, P. W.; Bailar, J. C.; and Polansky, M. "Crossover and Self-Controlled Designs in Clinical Research." *N Engl J Med* 310(1984):24–31.

Meinert, C. L. *Clinical Trials: Design, Conduct, and Analysis.* New York: Oxford University Press, 1986. A comprehensive text, somewhat skewed toward the big, multi-center clinical trial as opposed to the smaller effort, but covers most details and provides much practical wisdom about the difficult "conduct" step.

Sackett, D. L., and Gent, M. "Controversy in Counting and Attributing Events in Clinical Trials. *N Engl J Med* 301(1979):1410–12. Important issues in the difficult area of deciding who needs to be included at the time of outcome assessment.

Quasi-Experimental Designs

Campbell, D. T., and Stanley, J. C. *Experimental and Quasi-Experimental Designs for Research.* Boston: Houghton Mifflin Co., 1963. The original monograph.

Guyatt, G.; Sackett, D.; Taylor, D. W.; Chong, J.; Roberts, R.; and Pugsley, S. "Determining Optimal Therapy—randomized trials in Individual Patients." *N Eng J Med* 314(1986):889–92.

5

Data Collection, Management, and Analysis

MARIE McCORMICK AND
RICHARD C. WASSERMAN

Where to Start

Deciding What to Collect

The step before beginning to collect data is to consider exactly what information is needed to answer the research question and what is the most cost-effective way to obtain that data. It is worthwhile at this point to list specific data items (variables) and indicate a brief justification for the use of each in the study. Too often, beginning investigators start with a broad outline and engage in a time-consuming data collection process with the result that major portions of the data collection are unusable. The general basis for this approach is that, since reviewing the records or interviewing is going to be done anyway, it is not a major problem to collect the additional data, even if its usefulness is uncertain. Remember that every data item has its cost in terms of manpower to collect and enter it and of computer time to analyze it.

Another decision is type of data to be collected. These are:

- *Nominal*: People or events in unordered categories (e.g., black or white, dead or alive);
- *Ordinal*: People or events in ordered categories (e.g., 1 plus, 2 plus, 3 plus pitting edema);
- *Continuous*: Numbers are assigned or attached that have absolute meaning as a count or measurement by an objective scale (e.g., age, height, weight, score on the MCATs).

If possible, it is also a good idea to have some notion about the usual distributions for categorical (nominal or ordinal) variables and mean values and standard deviation for continuous variables. The reason for the latter recommendation is that such information is important in calculating sample size, which is discussed in Chapter 3. There are advantages and disadvantages to the different types of data. Generally, statistically significant differences can be achieved with smaller samples using continuous data than with nominal or ordinal data, but the latter are more often the kind of variables needed to make clinical decisions. The types of data to be collected depend on the question to be asked. For example, (and you must take this on faith or work it through with an experienced researcher), for a study of the association between physical activity in pregnant women and birthweight in a population with a mean birthweight of 3,100 g, a standard deviation of 300 g and a 10 percent low birthweight rate, 63 patients in each of two groups ("high" and "low" activity) would be sufficient to document a 300-g difference in birthweight, thus establishing an association, but 567 would be required to document a 50 percent difference (i.e., 10 versus 5 percent) in the rate of low birthweight infants. The latter might be more clinically relevant as the difference between 2,900 g and 3,200 g has less significance for reducing perinatal mortality and morbidity than the proportion of infants who are born small. This will become clearer after reading Chapter 3.

Most often clinical investigators collect data on individuals; however, studies may also be done using data based on groups or aggregates of individuals. For example, one might examine county mortality rates as a function of mean county income to attempt to document an association between socioeconomic status and the risk of dying. Alternatively, aggregate data might be used to estimate a characteristic of an individual (e.g., estimating income from the average income of the census tract in which the individual resides).

Since aggregate data are often readily available in routinely published sources, they are a convenient and accessible source of information to address many types of questions. In using such data, the investigator must be sensitive to two issues. One is called the *ecologic fallacy* and refers to the fact that associations based on aggregate data may not pertain to individuals. For example an individual may have an income substantially above or below his neighbors so that using an aggregate number may produce erroneous results. The other issue is that aggregate data may violate some of the assumptions underlying some statistical techniques, and consultation from a statistician may be in order.

Deciding How to Collect the Data

Once you have decided what data you need to answer your question, the next step is to decide the most appropriate source. In general, there are three basic types of data available for any study.

1. *Routine*: Data collected routinely for other purposes independent of the study (e.g., medical records, vital statistics, census data, hospital discharge abstracts, and national or local routine health surveys).
2. *Programmatic*: Data collected as part of a service program but not specifically related to a research project (e.g., patient–visit data, billing data, and vouchers).
3. *Primary*: Data specifically collected to address research questions (e.g., questionnaires and patient observations).

Once again, there are advantages and disadvantages to these three different types of data. Routinely collected data and programmatic data may be available for periods before or after the study and for subjects not directly involved, thus enhancing the investigator's ability to define comparison groups. In addition, since such data are collected under different auspices, the cost to the study may be relatively low compared to a new, study-specific data collection effort. A significant disadvantage to such data is the lack of control over the type and quality of data collected. Definitions may vary across sites or data collectors; coding conventions may also differ. Finally, with different persons collecting data for different purposes, the quality of the data may differ. With routinely collected data, the timing of availability is also not under the investigator's control but under the control of the agency. A different but analogous problem affects programmatic data; if the program does not succeed, the data will not be available.

Illustrations of these issues include:

- *Use of matched birth/infant death records.* The files are not complete until 1 year after the last birth in a year. That plus processing time means that such records are not available until at least 2 years after the year of the occurrence, and it might be longer with budget cuts.
- *Birthweight codes.* Although most states collect birthweight, coding conventions vary such that birthweight may be coded in exact grams, pounds and ounces, 250-g intervals or 500-g intervals.
- *Medical records.* Variability in different segments of the record have been documented. The chief complaint and diagnosis is usually listed; social data may be spotty and treatment information, especially counseling and advice, is almost always nonexistent.
- *Billing data.* Visit, diagnostic, and treatment information may be present only if the billing depends on it, so major disparities with medical records may exist.

All of this is not to preclude using such sources, but an argument for a careful review of the potential advantages and disadvantages as compared to a new data-collection effort. While the latter is likely to be more tailored to the research question and to be under greater control of the investigator, it may prove costly, and may limit the choice of experimental design.

Selecting Instrument/Data Collection Method

The selection of the specific data collection instrument or measures depends on several considerations.

Relevance to the Research Question

As noted earlier, data collection involves costs so that the inclusion of each piece of data should be carefully justified. For the beginner, it is often helpful to list the variables, and write out a justification for each.

Feasibility of Collection

Assessing the feasibility of different approaches to data collection is different for each study. If pre-existing records are to be used, those records must be accessible, and there has to be some assurance that the needed data have been collected in a form useful to the investigator. If primary data collection is contemplated, the researcher must investigate whether the numbers of appropriate subjects can be contacted within the time planned for the study and whether the subjects are likely to have the skills or knowledge necessary to complete the data-collection task. In addition, investigators must also ascertain whether they or their staff have the necessary skills. The logistics of contacting subjects and acquiring the data should be considered.

Finally, the types of data to be collected must be analyzable with the hardware and software available to the investigator.

Validity and Reliability of the Measure

Regardless of the method of data collection, the investigator must select measures that actually measure what the investigator wants (are valid) and do so consistently across subjects and observers (are reliable). In the laboratory, the analogous process would be the calibration of an instrument or procedure. The validity would be established by testing the ability of the instrument to detect a known standard substance or concentration. The reliability would be assessed through determining the variation in values produced by the instrument in repeated measure of the same standard. The purpose of this process is to reduce measurement error so that differences recorded among samples or subjects being studied reflect true differences and not just the instability of the instrument. Thus, if there was concern about accurate measures of alkaline phosphatase, the investigator would calibrate the measuring instrument against samples of known concentration throughout the range of the instrument with several repeats at each concentration.

Increasingly, clinical research involves data collection with interviews and observations derived from the social sciences methods. Examples would include IQ scores, behavior problem scales, attitudinal scales, social class, compliance measures, and the ability of screening tests to detect those with disease. It is important to understand assessing the validity and reliability of such measures, and this will be discussed later. As will be seen, using an established measure is preferred to starting from scratch. The full process will be described, however, in case it proves necessary. Also understanding some of the terms and procedures will help the investigator select from among existing instruments the one most appropriate for the study.

VALIDITY

Understanding how to assess validity involves a brief detour into some considerations from the theory of measurement. The thing that is to be measured is called a *construct*. A construct implies not only the content of the thing being measured but also what is known about its relationships with other events or constructs. In the case of the alkaline phosphatase example, the construct would involve not only the relationship of the test to the enzyme, but what is known about the composition of alkaline phosphatase and its behavior in the presence of normal or pathological conditions (e.g., growth and bony metastisis). Similarly, the construct of cognitive development would include not only the various domains of cognition (e.g., verbal skills, coordination, and quantitative skills), but also what is known to affect cognitive development (e.g., age, environmental stimulation, or neurological deficits).

This construct generates a universe of potential measures of the construct from which any single measure is considered to be a sample. Practically, the universe of potential measures is defined in several ways. Suppose, for example, the investigator wishes to develop a measure of easiness or difficulty in compliance with chronic medication regimens to predict situations in which compliance may be low. The first step might be to ask others who have performed research in compliance, so-called experts, to think about what might be included. Alternatively, the investigator might ask groups of patients to describe ways that help or limit their ability to take their medicines. This process tends to be iterative in that the responses gleaned from a group in one round are presented to the next group to assess the utility of the responses and to stimulate further discussion.

From the range of options thus generated, the investigator would then select the best way to measure the construct. This measure might be a single question, a number of questions that can be used as a scale, a single or series of observations or physical measurements, or a combination of questions and observations. In devising such a measure, it is well to get expert advice.

Whether the measure is developed de novo or the investigator is selecting from among established measures, the investigator is still faced with the question of whether the measure accurately reflects the construct to be studied. There are several levels at which this may be done; they are content (face) validity, criterion validity, and construct validity.

Content validity (or face validity) is a fancy way of saying, "It looks good to me." More specifically, on examination of the questions or observations in a measure, the items in the measure (either questions or observations) appear to reflect that which the investigator wishes to measure. Investigators may make their own assessment of the face validity or rely on the opinions of others. The fact, however, that a measure looks adequate does not mean that it will be appropriate for a given study. Without some indication of the prior use of the measure, it may prove difficult to assess whether or not the instrument can be administered in a way to obtain adequate information, can be used in populations like the potential study population, or is sensitive enough to measure differences of the type needed in the study.

Criterion validity is the next level of assessing validity and involves establishing the ability of a measure to predict performance on another measure of the same construct. Thus, for example, the investigator might be interested in the ability of a short-form test to predict performance on a more complex observational isntrument (e.g., the Peabody Picture Book Test to predict IQ as measured by more detailed testing).

A specific case of establishing criterion validity pertains to clinical medicine in the use of screening tests to assess clinical disease.

The validity of a screening test is assessed in terms of its sensitivity, specificity, and predictive values positive and negative. The criteria for developing a screening test and the definitions of the criteria are given in Figures 5.1 and 5.2, respectively. For the afficionados of acronyms, *sensitivity* or those with disease who test positive can be remembered as PID or positivity in disease; *specificity* or those without disease who are negative on the test as NIH or negativity in health. What is important to remember is that sensitivity and specificity are properties of the test (i.e., they should be the same across populations). The *predictive values* on the other hand are dependent on the prevalence of the disease in the population. For a test of given sensitivity and specificity, the lower the prevalence the more the positives will turn out to be false-positives.

A simple example using the formulas in Figure 5.2 will illustrate the latter point. Let us assume that we have a test that has a 90 percent sensitivity (i.e., the test is able to detect 90 percent of those with the disease). Let us also assume that the test has a 90 percent specificity (i.e., it correctly identifies 90 percent of those without disease). If the prevalence is 9 percent, in every 1,000 people, 90 (a and c) will have the disease and 910 (b and d) will not. Of the former, 81 (a) will be detected by the test, and 9 (c) will be missed. Similarly, of those without disease, 819 will be correctly identified,

---

1. Condition should be an important health problem
2. There should be an accepted treatment
3. Facilities for diagnosis and treatment should be available
4. The condition should have a recognizable latent or early symptomatic phase
5. There should be a suitable test or examination (cf below)
6. The test should be acceptable to the population
7. The natural history of the condition, including development is known
8. There should be an agreed policy on whom to treat
9. The cost of case-finding should be economically balanced in relation to possible expenditure on medical care as a whole
10. Case-finding should be a continuing process

FIGURE 5.1.   Criteria for Screening for Disease.

Source: J. M. G. Wilson, and G. Jungner, *Principles and Practice of Screening for Disease* (Geneva: World Health Organization, Public Health Paper no. 34, 1968).

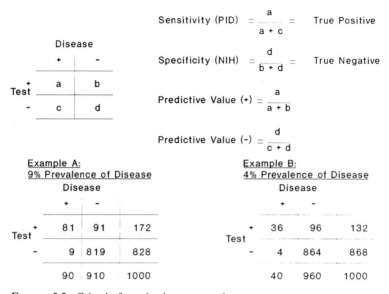

Sensitivity (PID) $= \dfrac{a}{a + c} =$ True Positive

Specificity (NIH) $= \dfrac{d}{b + d} =$ True Negative

Predictive Value (+) $= \dfrac{a}{a + b}$

Predictive Value (-) $= \dfrac{d}{c + d}$

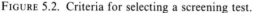

FIGURE 5.2. Criteria for selecting a screening test.

and 91 will be false positives. The test will be positive for 172 (a and b) subjects of whom 81 will have disease giving a predictive value positive for the test of 47.1 percent. Similarly, the test will be negative for 828 (c and d) people of whom 819 will be truly free of disease giving a predictive value negative of 98.9 percent.

What if the prevalence were 4 percent? The properties of the test, sensitivity and specificity, remain the same. Thus, of the 40 subjects with disease, 90 percent or 36 would be correctly identified and 4 would be missed. Of the 960 without disease 864 or 90 percent would be correctly noted, and 96 would be falsely identified as having disease. While the predictive value negative actually increases (864 of 868 or 99.5 percent), the predictive value positive has declined substantially (36 of 132 or 27.3 percent).

This principle of the trade-off between high sensitivity and of the risk of false positives has been incorporated into the development of receiver–operator characteristic (ROC) curves for selecting the optimal point for using a given test. For readers who are interested in a more complete description, the article by Griner (1981) provides a readable overview.

The earlier discussion would pertain to any situation in which the investigator is assessing the ability of any instrument to categorize the presence or absence of a characteristic, no matter how that characteristic is defined. When both the instrument and the standard are continuous variables, a correlation coefficient or regression coefficient is the appropriate measure. These are the standard parametric measures of association, and are referred to in Chapter 6. For example, if the investigator wished to assess the relationship of the Dubowitz test to the true gestational age, this would be done by correlating the Dubowitz score with gestational age. A correlation of 0.9 would suggest a high degree of correspondence; whereas a correlation of 0.3 would suggest little relationship between the two measures. In the latter case, the Dubowitz score might not be considered a valid measure of the gestational age.

Construct validity is the most difficult level of validity to assess. Considerations of establishing construct validity are the best argument for using established measures. Not only must the investigator assess whether the measure behaves internally as the construct predicts, but the relationships between this measure and other measures or observations are also what the construct would predict.

Internal consistency is a measure composed of a single item or observation and is relatively straightforward. If items are combined to yield a single measure or score of a construct, the investigator needs to establish that all the items are measuring the same thing. One way to assess this would be to split the items randomly into two halves, and correlate scores of one half with scores of the other. If the items were perfectly consistent, it should not matter which half of the scale was used and the correlation should be 1.0. Perfection is rarely achieved, however, and lesser values are acceptable. The most commonly used measure of internal consistency is an extension of the split-halves argument called *Cronbach's alpha*. It is usually expressed as a correlation coefficient, and generally values greater than 0.6 are considered acceptable. If the concern is how well individual items contribute to the overall score, the score on an individual item can be correlated with the overall score. Items that do not correlate well (i.e., < 0.6) with the total score might be dropped. The computer statistical package, Statistical Package for the Social Sciences (SPSS), has a routine that generates these measures.

Many scales or scores measure only a single, fairly narrow construct; others may measure constructs that are more complex. An example of the latter is the presence of subscales in many standard tests of cognitive development or IQ tests. If a construct is thought to have subcomponents, ideally the measure also ought to be divisible into subcomponents that relate to those predicted by the construct. The way this is tested is to determine the factor structure of the scale using factor analysis. Unless the investigator is familar with multivariate statistics, at this point it is time to call in the psychometrician. Determining factor structure is not simple. In assessing the reports of others, however, it is important to ask (1) do the items in each factor "make sense" (i.e., do they seem to have face validity)? and (2) are the factors internally consistent? For a layman's description of factor analysis, the reference by Stephen J. Gould on the Mismeasure of Man is particularly good (see suggested Readings at end of chapter). (It is also an excellent discussion on the use and abuse of IQ tests.)

Behavior in the real world. An investigator could develop a measure that met all the criteria tested so far and still not have a valid measure. The test is whether the measure behaves as you would expect it to behave; for example, the investigator might have a perfectly internally consistent measure for which high scores are thought to indicate "health." If, however, hospital inpatients scored high and those in health spa clubs scored low, the investigator might be very suspicious about what it was measuring (depending on your predjudices about health spa clubs).

More seriously, let us pursue the example of "health" for a moment. The construct "health" would predict a number of relationships: health should be better in higher social classes; it should be worse in people labeled "sick" by other measures; it should not vary by day of the week but might by season; and so on. Thus, establishing the construct validity would require a series of studies that would examine the behavior of these measures in a variety of populations in conjunction with other measures and in a variety of situations that permit assessing the sensitivity of the measure in reflecting changes in "health" in response to environmental changes that are known to affect "health" including experimental interventions. One way to assess construct validity is to examine the methodologic and other studies in which the measure has been used to examine questions of its usefulness in the specific research situation being planned. In addition, contacting those who developed the instrument may help in determining its appropriateness. Finally, a small pilot study (25 to 50 subjects) in groups similar to the one eligible for the study might be attempted. It is not only a good way to test the validity of the construct but also all other aspects of the study.

To do so the investigator would select a group to typify the situations in which the instrument was to be used. In the example of our measure of "health," the investigator might wish to include very sick and very well patients to assure that scores are really different between these groups (divergent validity or the ability to discriminate between/among groups known to be different). Among the sick patients, a variety of diagnoses might be included to assure that they would score similarly (convergent validity or ability to assess similarities across groups thought to be the same). For logistical purposes some examples of subjects who are difficult to interview or measure might be included (e.g., the handicapped, the mentally retarded, the illiterate, and non-English-speaking individuals). The analyses to be performed would parallel those outlined previously: internal consistency, factor analysis where appropriate, and comparison of scores or observations for different subgroups.

RELIABILITY

Even with a valid instrument, useful information may not be obtained equally well in all settings. Understanding the problem begins with the realization that every measure, no matter how precise, has an associated error (i.e., repeated measurement of exactly the same thing would produce different numbers). The closer these different numbers cluster around the true value, the lower the measurement error. The lower the measurement error, the more likely that differences in the measure across subjects represent true differences and not error.

Two sources of error in clinical measures are the subject and the observer. That is, the investigator may encounter variations in response from the same individual over time, and variations across observers with the same subject. Depending on the type of measure being used, there are a variety of sources of differences in response from the same subject. Performance may be affected by mood, fatigue, ability to concentrate, proximity to the event or duration of recall, learning over repeated administrations of the same items, or other intervening experiences that might increase or decrease scores. Similarly, without training and close supervision, different observers may also vary even when observing the same subject. The classic example is the differences in history and physical examination results among the attending, the resident, and the medical student. Besides experience, observers may vary in personality, understanding, and expertise with the tasks required, empathy with the subject, patience and tenacity with difficult subjects, and the combination of compulsivity and judgment that research data collection requires.

Several considerations pertain to selection of instruments to deal with reliability concerns. Clearly, measurements that are produced by machines that can be calibrated are likely to have less error than observations made by human beings. Asking a factual question produces more reliable responses than questions of attitude or belief. An extensive methodologic literature is available on different types of measures and sources of error. Some general references have been provided at the end of this chapter. In selecting a measure, the investigator should examine the literature with regard to both the specific measures/questions/observations and to the method of administration/data collection. In addition, it should be considered whether establishing the reliability of the measure may be required in the course of the planned study. Depending on the concerns generated by the literature and other previous experience, the investigator may need to assess the following:

1. *Intrarater reliability* refers to the degree to which the same interviewer/observer using the same measure obtains the same result on the same subject at two different points in time. This would clearly be most important when a measure is to be used more than once on the same subject in a before/after measure for an experiment or to measure changes over time in a longitudinal study.

2. *Interrater reliability* refers to the degree to which the different interviewers/observers using the same measure obtain the same result on the same subject. Interrater reliability is critical for combining data from different observers either within a site or across sites.

The basic method for establishing reliability is a repeated administration of the measure to a subject, either by the same or different observers at a time interval determined by the nature of the measure. Reliability is measured as the agreement between scores. The statistic is either a correlation coefficient for continuous or interval scores, or percent agreement for categorical data. In situations for which the categories are skewed so that the majority fall into one category, correction of the percent agreement for chance agreement is done using the Kappa statistic. An example is a test on which 90 percent of the population is "normal" and 10 percent "abnormal." On repeated measures, high agreement is likely as the population is likely to be "normal." Kappa would place more emphasis on the nonagreement and correct for chance agreement alone.

MODIFICATION

Because of the lack of instruments with well-established validity and reliability for a wide variety of clinical research situations, the clinical investigator is often faced with the question of the degree to which existing measures can be modified to the specific problem. In general, a strict constructionist point of view is probably safer (i.e., the instrument should be used as developed). Clearly, factual questions for which validity may be established in a relatively straightforward fashion are more amenable to modification than are attitudinal scales which should probably be used intact unless expert psychometric advice is available.

A particularly frequent situation in which modification is likely to be proposed is in obtaining diagnostic observations (e.g., physical exam or cognitive tests). There is always a trade-off between obtaining comparable data across subjects by standardizing the type and administration of observations and loss of information from detailed and creative observations with the special or unique patient (i.e., a trade-off between observations for research and for diagnostic purposes).

In considering any modification, the principles of establishing validity and reliability pertain. In other words, modification produces a new instrument that requires assessment.

The preceding discussion is not meant to dissuade the investigator from developing new measures if needed. Clearly, measuring what is needed for the research is preferred to measuring a tangential construct because an existing measure is available. When a new measure is required, the preceding discussion should provide an overview of the steps to be taken; however, when possible, the investigator, especially the neophyte, should search diligently for an appropriate, existing instrument. Established measures have the advantages that inappropriate items already might have been eliminated or modified by experience, the logistics of administration in various groups described, and data on validity and reliability available. Equally important is the fact that the use of the measure in the new study would make a contribution to the further documentation on that measure.

Data Management Procedures

Procedures Manual

All studies, regardless of size, require documentation of procedures, both as planned and as worked out in experience. This documentation can be described as a procedures manual that may vary in detail with the size of the study and the number of subjects involved. Nonetheless, regardless of the size or form, documentation of the following is essential:

1. Rules for determining subject eligibility/noneligibility for the study.
2. Format for recruiting subjects, explaining the study, getting informed consent, and managing refusals.
3. Definitions and sources of key data items.
4. Procedures for managing, coding, and entering data.
5. Changes in procedures over time.
6. Documentation of archiving policy.

While all of this may sound excessive for the relatively small study performed by a single investigator, one should be alert to the possibility of drift, which is the systematic changes in methods or coding over time. This can occur even with the most meticulous investigator and staff, because most clinical research projects may take 2–3 years between planning and final report. Changes in protocol and procedures occur with field experience, and may be critical to the interpretation of results. The discipline is worth it in the long run.

For large studies, the level of detail is a function of the number of observers and their independence from direct supervision by the principal investigator. For multi-site studies (i.e., studies in which observers are free agents with only periodic contact with the supervisor) or for lengthy studies in which staff turnover can be expected, these manuals may have to describe in detail the appropriate responses to each item, the degree to which unclear responses are accepted or can be probed, the acceptable probes, the management of potential problem situations (e.g., suspected child abuse by a lay home interviewer, the medical emergency), and the appropriate paperwork such as transmittal forms, daily logsheets to check productivity, travel reimbursement, and salary reports. Moreover, written records of all meetings may be needed to document decisions relevant to the research.

In planning the study and setting up procedures, some thought about the storage of data is worthwhile. One aspect of storage is ready access during the period of initial editing and analysis to check for errors. Another major concern, however, is the protection of confidentiality of the responses. Any research data that can be linked to individuals poses a threat of loss of confidentiality. Such linkages could be made if the medical record number is recorded on the data form, or if the data include a form on which study numbers used on computer files include subject names. While the study is being conducted such linkages are critical to record-keeping of the progress of the study. Records with such linkages should be kept in locked cabinets or file drawers to which only study staff have access. Once the study is complete, the investigator should give thought to whether the names will ever be needed again (i.e., for follow-up). If not, identifier files should be destroyed by removing face sheets with names or scrambling identifier numbers in the computer files.

Coding Manual

For larger data files, a coding manual may also be needed. It is often helpful even for small data sets. A coding manual specifies what is contained in the data file. It should contain:

- The full name of the variable.
- The abbreviated name in the data file, if appropriate.
- Location in file (for computer files this means specifying the field).
- Source (questionnaire, constructed from other variables).
- Allowable codes and definition of codes.

In addition, hard copies of key file specification programs and transformation programs are often handy for future reference. For example, respondent age is the variable of interest, but it is actually calculated from the date of birth and date of interview/observation. The exact algorithm for calculating respondent age should be saved and used to obtain the same number with each run. While this is a fairly simple example, documentation of data analytic decisions can save enormous grief and time when later analyses differ in the number of subjects because inclusion/exclusion rules were not clear, or when distributions differ (e.g., the number in each age group) because scoring algorithms were different.

Data Entry

How one enters data depends on the equipment and programs available, as well as the size and complexity of the data set. The advent of the microcomputer has only increased the options.

Many simple studies can be performed with hand counts, a calculator, and a reference text with the formulas of statistical texts, however, for many reasons, a more sophisticated approach is desirable. One is speed, although be forwarned that setting up any system takes about the same amount of thought and time on the first round. Editing, modifying, and replication are the major tasks enhanced by using a computer. A more important reason for computer use is accuracy; regardless of your proficiency with numbers, machine processing is more accurate and reproducible. A third reason is thoroughness, in that ease of data manipulation encourages exploration of the data. Finally, the amount of information available with machine processing is usually greater (e.g., exact chi square and p values).

A basic library, especially for microcomputers, should probably contain four types of programs: spreadsheet, data-base management, word-processing, and statistics.

A *spread-sheet program* is basically a large accounting sheet with cells into which words, numbers, or formulae may be entered. In addition, formulae manipulating the contents of two or more cells may also be used. The most current popular versions are the "-calc" programs (Vissicalc[R], Supercalc[R],) and Lotus 1-2-3[R]. These programs have been designed for budgets and projections, so that they are wonderful for grant proposals and financial reports. They also often interface with graphics packages which, with the right printer or screen/camera set up, may reduce audiovisual costs; however, since formulas can be entered, spread sheets can serve the same function as calculators with the advantage that the numbers and formulas can be visualized on the screen.

Data-base management programs can be thought of as fancy index card files. They are very useful for storing information that consists of many records in a common format (e.g., your reprint file) that may require sorting (e.g., by author, topic). In addition, these programs may also be used for data entry by creating forms on the screen that are similar to the investigator's data collection forms. They can even be set up to perform preliminary editing by specifying the values that are permissible. This helps to decrease typing errors in data entry. The most widely known of these programs and one of the most versatile is D-Base II or III[R].

Word-processing programs allow manipulation of text material. They have specific commands that insert, delete or rearrange material, change the format, paginate spacing between lines and paragraph, underline or boldface titles, and set up tabs for columns. With some of the new graphics packages, it is even possible to insert illustrations or drawings. For the most common uses of most researchers (grant proposals and papers), the initial entry of the document into the word-processing program is about the same as with an electric typewriter. What is vastly simplified and neater is the insertion of the co-investigator's or chairman's scathing comments into the second draft, replacing the arduous work of cutting, pasting, lining up, and photocopying that occurred in the past.

Secretaries (and chairmen) encourage familiarity with word-processing programs for obvious reasons. For the proficient typist, however, they do make drafting more efficient. In addition, for the less proficient typist, they may make programming or using large statistical programs on a mainframe easier in that instructions can be written and edited in the word-processing program. There are almost hundreds of suitable programs.

Statistical packages vary from those in books with programs that can be entered by hand to very powerful, comprehensive packages. All of the major well-known packages are, or shortly will be, available for suitably equipped microcomputers (e.g., SPSS, SAS, and BMDP). In addition, many programs designed to go with spread-sheet programs for economic forecasting in business are powerful analytic tools. The choice of package involves cost of equipment and software, the size and complexity of data sets, the investigator's own statistical sophistication, and access to a mainframe computer. For most departmental or divisional uses, however, the trend appears to be to purchase a powerful microcomputer and use of a mainframe-like package (e.g., SPSS). For more modest needs, there are a wide variety of programs. The most difficult subroutine, however, is often the one of most interest to clinicians; namely, cross-tabulations two by two or larger tables). Not all micros have the memory to array numbers of such form. For this reason, the chi-square or tabulation program should be checked carefully.

Of greatest importance in selecting hardware (machines) and software (programs) are the following factors:

Compatability among machines being used by collaborators, between machines and programs that are supposed to interface (e.g., the word-processing program in the microcomputer being used as a terminal to access a mainframe) and among programs. No time is saved if the investigator and the secretary are using different word-processing programs. In this regard, the word compatible should be viewed with caution when applied to machines; achieving compatability may require more reprogramming skills to modify software than most of us possess. Reviews in computer magazines often benchmark machines against complex programs to assess this. In addition, many newer programs now come with instructions on how to modify files to fit.

Transportability between different types of machines and programs. Compatability may help but does not guarantee communication among different computing units or programs. For example, one may plan to analyze the data on a microcomputer, but the data set may prove to be too large, necessitating transfer to a mainframe. Another common situation is having collected the data using one program (e.g., D-Base III) and wishing to analyze the data with another (e.g., SPSS). Alternatively, what do you do if you have the data on an IBM and your co-investigator has a MacIntosh? Machine-specific software definitely inhibits transport (i.e., software specific to a single machine in a unique language). One way to get around some of the differences in equipment is to use programs that rely on transportable programming languages like ASCII. Information may be transported from one machine to another in ASCII, and reformatted to local use.

One final piece of advice. A generalist must rely on consultants in other clinical areas; cultivate reliable consultants in research design, instrumentation and measurement, methods for collecting data, and data hardware and software.

Data Analysis

This section will provide an overall approach to data analysis, including an overview of basic categories of analysis, a brief discussion of some of the more standard statistical and epidemiologic tools for testing associations, and a review of some common pitfalls in data analysis.

There is no magic to statistics. Statistics are a set of techniques used for describing, analyzing, and interpreting data. Descriptive statistics are those used to characterize particular groups. The process of translating empirical observations from single studies into broader generalizations is called *statistical inference*, and is accomplished using statistical tests of significance. Because excellent discussions of statistical inference and hypothesis testing and the formulas for calculating statistical tests are available in numerous statistics books, they will not be included in this section.

The modern clinical investigator should use a computer to perform data analysis. Questions about the analysis of data from a specific study should always be discussed with either a statistician or with a colleague who has expertise in statistical analysis and some familiarity with the study.

An Overview of Data Analysis

A plan for data analysis should exist before the data are gathered. One approach is to set up all the tables for the presentation of results during the planning stages of a study. The investigator will then only have to fill in the blanks after the data are gathered. This will also decrease the likelihood of omitting necessary or gathering unnecessary data.

The nature of the analysis is determined by the type of research being performed and the types of variables being used. The typology of research designs has already been discussed in Chapter 4.

The reader should remember that variables might be categorized in different ways such as categorical or nominal, ordinal, ranked, or numerical (see Figure 5.3). *Nominal* data are variables whose values are categories or names. They may be dichotomous

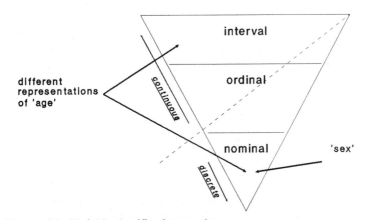

FIGURE 5.3. Variable classification overlap.
SOURCE: D. G. Kleinbaum, and L. L. Kupper. *Applied Regression Analysis and Other Multivariable Methods*. (Boston: Duxbury Press, 1978).

(e.g., alive versus dead) or have several classifications (e.g., race, blood type). *Ordinal variables* have an implicit and logical order or structure, such as a rating of personal health with responses of poor, fair, good, or excellent. Although the ratings have an inherent logic, the intervals between classes are not assumed to be equal. *Ranked variables* have an order within a given group. An example of a ranked variable is a group of children ranked by height from shortest to tallest. *Numerical variables* are numbers. They can be *discrete*, such as the number of children in a family, or *continuous*, such as height or weight. Discrete variables can be treated statistically as though they were continuous, but often yield results that do not make strict biologic sense (e.g., average family size of 2.5 children).

Variables can also be classified according to their relation to one another. Common classifications are independent, dependent, control, and confounding. *Independent variables*, also called manipulated or treatment variables, are so named because they are independent of the outcome itself. They are presumed to cause or influence the outcome. *Dependent variables*, also called outcome or response variables, are so named because they are dependent on the independent variables. The outcome thus depends on how the independent variables either occur or are manipulated. *Control variables*, also called background variables, are so named because they need to be controlled, randomized, or held constant in order to neutralize their effects. Common examples are age, sex, and race. *Confounding variables*, which are discussed in more detail later, are independent variables that distort the magnitude of association between another independent variable and a dependent variable.

Initial Descriptive Analysis

Assuming that all the data have been entered into a computer data file, the initial step is to analyze them descriptively. Through a descriptive analysis, the investigator ensures that the data have been correctly recorded and digested by the computer. Furthermore, each variable becomes more familiar to the investigator and can be used to provide a basis for more complex analyses.

Each variable needs to be checked to ensure that the recorded values are plausible. Inspection may reveal the presence of *outliers*;

that is, individual observations that are extreme with respect to the rest of the data. They are important because they can exert a large influence on the results of an analysis, especially when sample sizes are small. The investigator must first make sure that an outlier is not the result of a recording error. If it appears to be, it should be corrected, or if this is not possible, treated as missing data (see later). If an outlier does not appear to represent a mistake, it can be included in the analysis, with an awareness of its possible effects and distortions.

For each variable it is common to find one or more cases with missing values. Missing data are not usually a problem as long as they are few in number. These cases can usually be omitted without affecting the results. If, however, there are large numbers of missing values (e.g., >20 percent of the sample) the possibilities for error increase and excluding cases may distort the results. When this occurs it is best to discuss the options with a biostatistician who is familiar with the study.

Categorical variables are best examined using frequency distributions. These are lists of the frequencies with which each category or value of the variable occur in the data, usually accompanied by the proportion (number with the particular value divided by the total number observed) represented. For ordinal variables, frequency distributions can provide a *median* (that value that separates the observations into two halves), as well as other important division points, such as the twenty-fifth or seventy-fifth percentiles. Visual representations such as bar graphs and pie charts are especially useful for describing variables with multiple categories, and they can usually be generated with computer statistical packages.

Numerical variables should also be examined using frequency distributions. Histograms (i.e., bar-type diagrams that depict the distribution) should be generated to reveal whether it is symmetrical or skewed. Since many statistical tests theoretically require a Normal or Gaussian distribution, it is important to know if this assumption is being met. When frequency distributions are not symmetrical, often they can be mathematically transformed (e.g., converted logarithmically) in order to make the statistical techniques valid.

Numerical variables must also be characterized with a measure of central tendency (mean, mode, or median) and a measure of distribution or spread. The *mean* is the average value, calculated by summing the individual values and dividing by the total number of the group ($x = \Sigma x / n$). The mean is the most commonly used measure of central tendency because it is amenable to mathematical manipulation. It is, however, greatly affected by outlier observations and asymmetry in the distribution. The *median*, defined previously, is unaffected by outliers and might be the more appropriate measure when a distribution is skewed. The *mode*, or value that occurs most frequently, reveals the most typical value for that variable.

The simplest measure of distribution or spread is the *range*, defined as the highest minus the lowest value. Unfortunately the range is extremely sensitive to outliers, tends to increase with the total number of observations, and is difficult to treat mathematically. The *variance*, defined as the average of the squares of the deviations about the mean $[V(x) = \Sigma(x - x)^2/(n - 1)]$, is quite amenable to mathematical manipulation but has the disadvantage of being expressed as the square of the units of the original observations. The *standard deviation* is the most commonly employed measure of distribution. Calculated as the square root of the variance $\mathrm{SD}(x) = \sqrt{V(x)} = \sqrt{\Sigma(x - x)^2/n - 1}$, the standard deviation is amenable to mathematical treatment and is expressed in the same units as the original observations.

Having generated initial descriptive statistics for the variables, it is useful to perform crosstabulations on categorical variables of interest. *Crosstabulations* are joint frequency distributions of cases according to two or more categorical variables. The simplest example of a crosstabulation is the so-called two by two contingency table. For example the investigator might examine the study population by both race (nonwhite versus white) and sex. Looking at this two by two table would provide the investigator with an idea of the distributions of each sex by race.

A series of crosstabulations, which need not necessarily be limited to two columns and two rows, can provide the investigator with clues of the various associations in the data. *Scattergrams*, plots of two numerical variables on an x and y axis, are useful for visually representing relationships among numerical variables. An example is a plot of hematocrit by age. These and other exploratory techniques also can help to generate other questions hypotheses from descriptive studies.

Statistical Tests of Significance

Most clinical studies, however, are either comparative or experimental, as described previously. In these types of studies, the researcher is investigating possible associations of one or more independent variables with one or more dependent (outcome) variables and, therefore, these associations must be assessed. The most commonly used tools for assessing associations are significance tests. An overview of the tests discussed later can be seen in Table 5.1. Calculation of a statistical test results in a probability or p value, which can be defined as the likelihood that the observed pattern of independent and dependent variables could have been observed by chance. For example, a p value of $<.01$ for a difference in outcomes between treatment and control groups in a clinical trial of a drug means that there is less than a 1 percent chance that the observed difference between the groups is due to chance alone.

By convention, an *alpha* value of .05 (or occasionally .01) is arbitrarily selected as a cutoff for defining statistical significance, with all p values below alpha reflecting significant associations between variables. Alpha therefore defines the likelihood of an error in the study's apparent associations (i.e., the chance that the associations found to be statistically significant are not true). This error has been called *type I error*.

Type II error is the error of failing to detect a true difference between two compared groups. To guard against type II error, an investigator who finds no significant difference in a crucial test of a study hypothesis should calculate the *power* or likelihood of finding a true difference if in fact one existed. Formulas and nomograms for calculating statistical power are available in statistics text books and in journal articles on this subject.

The most basic analyses carried out are bivariate (i.e., tests of the relationship between two variables). In general, if both independent and dependent variables are numerical, the best test is the correlation coefficient (Pearson's r). The *correlation coefficient*, derived from the process of linear regression, is an estimate of the

TABLE 5.1. Overview of Statistical Tests of Significance

Test	Variables Dependent	Variables Independent	Comments
Correlation coefficient (Pearson's *r*)	Numerical	Numerical	Parametric, simple linear regression
Correlation coefficient (Kendall, Spearman)	Ranked	Ranked	Nonparametric
t Test	Numerical *or* Dichotomous	Dichotomous Numerical	Parametric
Analysis of variance	Numerical *or* Categorical	Categorical Numerical	Parametric, more than 2 categories
Chi-square	Categorical	Categorical	Nonparametric
Fisher's exact test	Categorical	Categorical	Nonparametric, for small sample sizes (n < 20)
Multiple regression	Numerical	Numerical or Categorical	Parametic, used to control for confounding variables
Multivariate discriminant analysis	Categorical	Numerical or Categorical	Parametric, used to control for confounding variables
Nonparametric tests (e.g., Sign test, rank sum test)	Categorical, ordinal, or ranked	Categorical, ordinal, or ranked	Nonparametric

strength of the relationship between the dependent and independent variables. Values greater than 0.5 are generally viewed as strong, and a *p* value is calculated with the correlation. In using the test it is assumed that both variables have Normal distributions. Statistical tests in which particular (usually Normal) distributions are assumed are called *parametric tests*. If the assumption in this case is violated, the investigator might use the test after transforming the data as described previously. Alternatively, the investigator could use a nonparametric, "ranked" correlation test (Kendall's or Spearman's correlation). An example of an appropriate use of the correlation coefficient test is to test the relationship between height and serum creatinine in a group of patients.

Often an investigator wants to test the association between a numerical dependent variable (e.g., systolic blood pressure) and a categorical independent variable (e.g., whether or not a patient in a clinical trial was treated with propranolol). In this case, the appropriate test is the *t-test*. Use of the t-test assumes a Normal distribution. In some studies, patients may serve as their own controls, and a different form of the t-test is needed. If, for example, a group of hypertensive patients were given either propranolol or placebo for 1 month and then switched over to the other treatment in the second month, the special version of the t-test, known as the *paired t-test* would be needed.

The t-test is also appropriate if the dependent variable is categorical and dichotomous (e.g., dead or alive) and the independent variable is numerical (e.g., birthweight). Thus if an investigator was performing a study to assess the association of postneonatal mortality and birthweight, one could also use the t-test. If the independent or dependent variable is categorical but has more than two categories (e.g., dead, alive with handicap, alive without handicap), the appropriate statistical test is the *analysis of variance* (ANOVA).

When both the independent and dependent variables are categorical, the appropriate statistical test is the *chi-square test*. In a chi-square of the association of two dichotomous variables, a two by two table will be created. The values in each of the four cells represent counts of the cases that fit the criteria as determined by the columns and rows. The chi-square test is very sensitive to sample size. For small samples, where the expected value for any cell is less than five, another test, known as *Fisher's exact test*, should be used instead of the chi-square.

After the investigator performs a series of bivariate analyses, it is often useful to draw a diagram representing the associations that have been found. If, for example, the two independent variables, age and education, are both significantly correlated with the dependent variable compliance with medication use, it is necessary to see to what extent age and education are associated with one another. If the apparent association between age and compliance can be accounted for by education, it is said that education "confounds" that association. Failure to detect *confounding variables* can lead the investigator to incorrect conclusions.

There are two strategies for dealing with potential confounding variables. One strategy, favored by epidemiologists, is called *stratification*. In stratification, the investigator tests for the association between independent and dependent variables in subsamples that have been stratified in terms of the potential confounding variable. For example, the investigator could compare the strength association between age and compliance in a low education group with that found in a high education group.

A second strategy for dealing with possible confounding variables is the use of multivariate statistical techniques. These techniques allow investigators to test associations between two variables while simultaneously controlling for other variables. Two examples will be briefly mentioned here. One is known as *multiple regression analysis*. Multiple regression is an elaborate version of the simple correlation test mentioned earlier. In calculating a simple correlation coefficient, a linear regression is actually performed. In multiple regression, a series of linear regressions are performed according to certain prestated guidelines. Multiple regression is an appropriate technique to use when the dependent variable is a continuous one. If the dependent variable is a dichotomous categorical variable, then a technique called *multivariant discriminant analysis* can be used. Both of these methods and other multivariate techniques are frought with potential problems, and should not be used by the investigator without the assistance of a biostatistician.

Another important group of statistical tests are the *nonparametric tests*. Most of the tests discussed previously are parametric, requiring estimates of parameters (e.g., mean, standard deviation), certain types of variables (continuous), and making assumptions about the underlying distribution of the data (e.g., normality). Often, however, the data to be analyzed are not appropriate for parametric testing (e.g., categorical), or the assumptions required for parametric methods are not easily satisfied. Nonparametric tests make no assumptions about the shape of the underlying data distribution. Several of the tests already mentioned, the Kendall and Spearman rank correlations, the chi-square test, and the Fisher's exact test, are nonparametric tests. Numerous other tests are available for a variety of situations. All involve either categorical, ordinal, or ranked variables. All can be used on relatively small samples. The investigator who wants to use them to analyze data will need to consult one of the cited text books devoted to these tests and also discuss them with a biostatistician.

Alternatives to Significance Testing

Exclusive reliance on tests of significance in data analysis can mislead the researcher, because test results are in part a function of sample size, and because P values give little information on the actual magnitude of an association. When sample sizes are very large, associations of small magnitude or minimal clinical importance may yield significant P values. When sample sizes are small, strong associations might fail to achieve statistical significance. Two commonly used alternatives to significance testing are confidence intervals, and risk or odds ratios.

A *confidence interval* gives the calculated limits, at an arbitrarily defined level of confidence (usually 95 or 90 percent), within which the true value of an estimated parameter is likely to occur. They are especially useful in comparing treatment outcomes. Whereas significance tests lend themselves to yes or no interpretations of association, confidence intervals are descriptive. For example, in a small clinical trial comparing treatment protocols for neuroblastoma, the researcher finds a mean difference in remission rates between protocols A and B of 25 percent with a 95 percent confidence interval of 0 to 50 percent. This means there is a 95 percent likelihood that the true mean difference between treatments falls between no difference and protocol A being 50 percent better. Because the 95 percent confidence interval includes 0 percent, this difference in remission rates would not be statistically significant at the .05 level, and the protocol might be rejected by a naive researcher. Examination of the confidence interval allows the researcher to see that protocol A most likely has a positive and potentially large advantage over B. An increase in sample size will narrow the width of the confidence interval. A more complete discussion of confidence intervals, including formulas for their calculation, can be found elsewhere (Armines and Zeller 1979).

Risk and *odds ratios* represent a second alternative to significance testing. These are epidemologic measures of association calculated from two by two tables (see Figure 5.4). The *risk ratio* is calculated as $a/(a + b) \div c/ (c + d)$. Commonly it refers to the risk of a disease among those exposed to an agent compared to the risk in those unexposed. Thus a risk ratio of 1.0 indicates equal risk, and therefore no association.

A related calculation is the *odds ratio*, used when the data in the two by two table are derived from a case–control study. The odds ratio is calculated as $ad \div bc$, and closely approximates the risk ratio. The risk ratio and odds ratio express the magnitude of association between an independent variable and the dependent variable. The values of these measures are not affected by sample size and may be considered even when p values are not statistically significant.

It is possible to calculate confidence intervals for the risk ratio and odds ratio, and these are affected by sample size. If the confidence interval includes 1.0, the investigator can assume that the association is questionable, but the upper limit of the interval should also be considered in evaluating the strength of the association. Discussions of the risk ratio and odds ratio are often absent from statistics texts. They are more fully discussed in texts focusing on epidemiologic techniques.

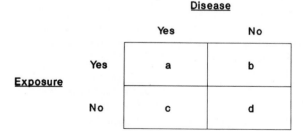

FIGURE 5.4. Two by two table.

Common Pitfalls

Common pitfalls in data analysis are as follows: First there is the failure to analyze data on those individuals who were eligible for the study but who, for some reason, were excluded. If such an analysis is not carried out, the external validity or generalizability of the study is threatened. Investigators need to compare those subjects included in the study with those who declined participation on as many variables as possible. If it can be shown that the two groups do not differ significantly on any of the known variables, the sample population that has been studied can be assumed to be representative.

Second is the use of multiple tests of significance (e.g., a series of t tests) when comparing two groups. With each test of significance, the likelihood increases of finding a significant association by chance alone. This problem can be dealt with in several ways. One way is to forego unnecessary hypothesis testing. A second way is to correct for multiple testing by using a smaller alpha value for judging "significance." Methods for adjusting alpha values can be found in statistics texts or in articles devoted to this subject. A third way is to make use of a multivariate technique as discussed earlier in order to provide a unified analysis that simultaneously incorporates the many associations among the variables.

Finally there is insufficient sample size, as discussed previously under research design. A sufficient sample size is important to avoid a type II error.

In keeping with the purpose of this manual, this discussion has touched on some of major issues in data analysis. The investigator is encouraged to use the reference list, seek advice from research colleagues, and make appropriate use of consultants in order to enhance skills in this area. In many ways, analysis is the most enjoyable part of research. It is also the most risky and can be the most frustrating. An inadequate or incorrect analysis can produce worthless or even misleading results from soundly collected data. The investigator has an intellectual and moral responsibility to assure the excellence of the data analysis. After all the time, energy, and expense of performing the study to collect the data, this part should provide the pay off.

When and How to Work With a Statistician

Finding a statistician to work with might not be easy. The biostatistics department of the nearest medical school or school of public health is a good place to start. An experienced colleague who has performed clinical research might be able to recommend someone. The ideal statistician is someone who has worked on projects similar to the one the researcher is planning. Clinician researchers and biostatisticians often have problems communicating, and it is important to find someone accustomed to talking to clinicians and who can understand why and how the research is being undertaken.

The time to talk to a statistician is *before* the data are gathered. It is best to seek advice when designing the research methods. A brief discussion of study plans and procedures can prevent a simple oversight that might compromise the study results or save the expense of gathering unnecessary data. If the investigator cannot find a statistician for this purpose, a social scientist, research psychologist, sociologist, or a physician experienced with clinical research can often provide the same service.

A beginning investigator with access to a computer statistics program can conduct the analysis alone. This is, in fact, the best way to learn the use of statistical packages and computer hardware. Until the investigator is quite experienced, however, it is better to make extensive use of a statistician to discuss analyses and results.

Finally, it is useful to make expectations about the statistician's role in the study very explicit. Many statisticians work on a consulting basis and expect only remuneration. Others might want to be included as co-author in presentations or publications that result from the study. It is best to make these arrangements clear at the outset.

Communication of Results

A well conducted and well analyzed research project is meaningless if no one ever hears about it. The scientific enterprise is a cumulative one, and proper communication of the investigator's results is crucial. Communication of results can take place in several forms. Typically, a short abstract is submitted for potential presentation at a scientific meeting. If the abstract is selected, the investigator must prepare a short presentation. Ultimately, however, the investigation should be presented into the scientific literature by being published in a peer-reviewed journal. Several aspects of this process will be discussed.

Writing an Abstract

In an abstract, the investigator needs to distill the entire project, from conception to conclusions, into approximately 200 words. Although the temptation might exist to dwell on the importance of the research and to speculate on its conclusions, there is little space for this aspect in the study. The investigator needs to concentrate on the study methods and the results.

A maximum of two to three sentences should be used to introduce the rationale for and goal of the investigation, followed by a brief discussion of the methods. The investigator should review the nature of the population under study, how subjects were recruited, what proportion declined to participate, and whether or not those who participated were different from those who did not. Next threre should be a description of what data were gathered outlining the important variables and how they were gathered. At the conclusion of the methods section, the general analytic strategy should be outlined.

In the results section, the characteristics of the study population should be described with the focus on those results most central to the study. There should be enough discussion of results to deal with obvious questions that might arise in the interpretation of the data.

The conclusion should contain one sentence to summarize the important findings and perhaps another to mention the ultimate relevance of the work.

Presentations

If the investigator is fortunate enough to have an abstract accepted, the presentation must then be prepared. Presentations at scientific meetings are generally 10 minutes long, with an additional 5 minutes allotted for discussion. They run on an extremely tight schedule, and moderators frown on individuals who go over their allotted time.

The challenge of presenting a research study in 10 minutes' time is perhaps greater than that of writing an abstract. Since a major purpose of presenting the work is to obtain feedback from individuals interested in the subject, the study must be presented in appropriate detail.

As in the abstract, the introduction and rationale for the study should be kept to a minimum. There need be little or no literature review. Once again, the presenter needs to concentrate on the methods and results sections.

Slides are a must but improperly prepared slides can detract from a presentation. Slides need to be simple, easy to read, and self explanatory. A general rule is to use approximately one slide per minute of presentation. A typical format for slides might be as follows: one slide to state the goals of the research, one to describe how they were selected for the study, one to outline the research design, one to list the variables and data collected, five for presenting the results, and one to state the study conclusions. In the presentation, the investigator might indulge in commenting on the results. It should be remembered, however, that there will be another 5 minutes of questions and answers at the conclusion of the presentation.

To be comfortable with the presentation, it is crucial that the presenter practice ahead of time with the actual slides to be used and a pointer. There is no better way to find out about the problems of a presentation than to present it several times to colleagues at the home base. This will allow for appropriate timing of the presentation and for the presenter to anticipate the questions that will be asked. It is often useful to prepare several extra slides to help explain those anticipated questions.

Publication

Publication of study results in a peer-reviewed journal is usually the ultimate goal of research. It is a sobering fact that over half of all presentations at scientific meetings are not published within the next several years. Although there are a number of reasons for this, a major factor is that the preparation of a manuscript for publication is a very exacting and time-consuming process; however, much of this process can be accomplished as the study is designed and implemented.

The elements of a good journal article might vary from study to study, but in general the following are necessary. There should be a clear and succinct statement of the problem being addressed. A review of relevant literature, organized conceptually rather than chronologically, should follow. Next the author should outline the rationale and specific goals and hypotheses of the project. Following this introduction there should be a methods section that includes a detailed description of study methods and addresses the rationale for the particular methods chosen. There should be a detailed description of the study design, study population, data-gathering instruments and techniques, and all study procedures. The methods section should also contain an outline for the proposed analysis of the data.

The results section should contain all relevant results that are often best communicated in the form of tables or figures. If these are used, they should be entirely self explanatory and not redundant with the text.

Following the results is a discussion section in which those conclusions that are supported by the study's results should be drawn. A discussion of the limitations of the study methods and results is appropriate. Comparisons with the results of similar studies should be made. Although a certain amount of speculation is permissible, it should be minimized. Recommendations for future research in the area of investigation are also appropriate.

In general the article should be written with a specific journal in mind. This is important for the particular audience that is being addressed and for any stylistic conventions that a particular journal might require.

Some time after submission of the article, the author will receive the comments of the reviewers. The article is rarely accepted as is. More commonly it is either accepted contingent on certain revisions, or is rejected. Since only a minority of submitted articles are selected for publication in most journals, a rejection should be viewed as an opportunity to improve the article, rather than as an insult.

In making revisions and resubmitting the article it is wise to address the suggested revisions by number in a letter to the editor, pointing out where in the new text they have been incorporated. If for some reason a suggested revision can or should not be made, this should be explained in detail to the editor.

If an article is rejected, it is wise to include as many of the suggestions made by the reviewers as possible in preparing a new draft. It is likely that the reviewers for the next journal to which you submit the article would react similarly to the original manuscript. Providing them with a manuscript that has benefited from review will increase the chances for acceptance.

Suggested Readings

Carmines, E. G., and Zeller, R. A. *Reliability and Validity Assessment.* Sage University Papers on Quantitative Applications in the Social Sciences 07-017. Beverly Hills: Sage Publications, 1979.

Fowler, F. *Survey Methods.* Beverly Hills: Sage Publications.

Hollander, M., and Wolfe, D. A. *Nonparametric Statistical Methods.* New York: John Wiley and Sons, 1973.

Gould, Stephen J. *The Mismeasure of Man.* New York: Norton, 1981.

Griner, P. F. et al. "Selection and Interpretation of Diagnostic Tests and Procedures." *Ann Intern Med* 94(1981):453.

Madron, T. W.; Tate, C. N.; and Brookshire, R. G. *Using Microcomputers in Research.* Sage University Paper in Quantitative Applications in the Social Sciences 07-52. Beverly Hills:Sage Publications, 1985.

Schrodt, P. A. *Microcomputer Methods for Social Scientists.* Sage University Paper on Quantitative Applications in the Social Sciences 07-040. Beverly Hills: Sage Publications, 1984.

Schwartz, W., and Hammer, L. "Use of Microcomputers in the Division of General Pediatrics." *Pediatrics* 71(1983):328.

Siegel, S. *Nonparametric Statistics for the Behavioral Sciences.* New York: McGraw-Hill, 1956.

Simon, R. "Confidence Intervals for Reporting Results of Clinical Trials." *Ann Intern Med* 105(1986):429–35.

6

Pragmatics

ANNE K. DUGGAN

> A foundation is a large body of money completely surrounded
> by people who want some. So get in line. . .
>
> (Dwight MacDonald)

More likely than not, the process of formulating the research
question will generate visions of the "ideal" study to answer it. The
"real world," however, rarely offers the opportunity to employ the
perfect research strategy. Financial and ethical considerations place
constraints on what is feasible. As a consequence, the researcher is
compelled to restructure the ideal study design. The challenge in
this restructuring is to maintain scientific integrity while conform-
ing to ethical mandates and staying within the temporal and economic bounds of feasibility. Collaboration can be a useful tool for
expanding the latter. This chapter describes the pragmatic aspects
of research: projecting and minimizing research costs, securing
funding, assuring compliance with ethical standards for research
involving human subjects, and developing collaborative arrangements.

Projecting Costs

Virtually all funding groups require a budget and justification as part of the research proposal; however, research costs should be projected as part of planning even if the study is small and not anticipated to require outside funding. There are at least two reasons for this. First, by considering the time, effort, and materials required to complete each step in the research process, the researcher is less likely to be compromised by unanticipated resource needs midstudy. Second, comparison of alternative research methods allows development of the most cost-efficient plan.

The Public Health Service research grant application budget requirements are illustrative of those for most funding sources and provide a good framework for projecting costs for both clinical and health services research. Costs are categorized into nine groups: personnel, consultant costs, equipment, supplies, travel, patient care costs, alterations and renovations, consortium/contractual costs, and other expenses. A detailed budget is required for the first 12 months of the research; for subsequent years, only the total request for each category is required. This is usually accompanied by an indication of the anticipated annual increase in personnel costs and a brief justification of any significant increase in any expense category over the first 12-month budget period. Table 6.1 displays the types of information and level of detail expected by most funding agencies.

The vast majority of research funding is awarded to institutions, not individuals. Assuming the researcher is applying for funding through an institution (e.g., medical school, hospital, or professional association), administrative staff should be consulted to provide needed information for calculating budget needs, (e.g., fringe benefit rate for personnel and indirect cost rate) and to assure that the final product conforms to institutional regulations. In large organizations, the internal budget review process can take up to 2 weeks, and sometimes longer, even if there are no problems. For this reason experienced researchers often find it more time efficient to first develop the research plan in general, prepare the budget, send it off for departmental and institutional administrative approval, and then write the final research plan while the budget section is being reviewed.

TABLE 6.1. Categories of Expense and level of Detail
Required in Research Proposal Budgets

Category	Information to be Included
Personnel	For each individual involved in the project: name, position, function, hours/week or percent effort, salary, fringe benefits.
Consultant costs	For each consultant who has agreed to serve as such: name, institutional affiliation, services to be performed, number of days of consultation, anticipated rate of compensation, travel, per diem and related cost.
Equipment	Separate listing of each item with a unit acquisition cost of $500 or more.
Supplies	Itemized listing by type (e.g., glassware, office supplies, postage).
Travel	Number and purpose of trips, destinations, number of travelers.
	Separate itemization for domestic vs. foreign.
	Detailed justification for foreign travel.
Patient care costs	For each medical institution to be reimbursed for in- or outpatient charges incurred as part of the research: name, amount requested, basis on which amount calculated (e.g., a rate previously negotiated by the hospital and the DHHS), number of patient days or visits, cost/day or/ visit, cost/test or treatment.
Alterations and renovations	Itemized listing by type (e.g., painting, repairs, installation of partitions); basis for calculating costs (e.g., contractor's detailed estimate).
Consortium/ contractual costs	For each consortium and major contractual arrangement, the total amounts requested for direct and indirect costs should be accompanied by itemized budgets containing the same categories as for the budget as a whole.
Other expenses	Itemized listing, unit cost and justification of all other expenses (e.g., books, computer time, rentals, equipment maintenance, research subject reimbursement for travel, lodging, subsistence), minor fee-for-service contracts.

The scope of internal administrative budget review in general is limited to a check of completeness, arithmetic accuracy, and conformance with institutional guidelines. It is not concerned with the rationale underlying the volume and types of resource need projections. The soundness of projections is the responsibility of the researcher. Personnel needs are best estimated by considering the skills and time required to perform each task in the research process. Where lack of experience precludes an informed estimate, the researcher is well advised to consult with colleagues who have such experience and if at all possible, to conduct a pilot test of study procedures. With many data collection tasks, 95 percent of the work proceeds routinely, comprising about half of the staff's time and effort. The last 5 percent, however, consumes an equal amount of time. Murphy's Law ("If something can go wrong, it will.") is operative at some point in most research. A pilot test of all study procedures provides invaluable information for estimating the personnel, materials, and time needed for their successful completion and helps the investigator to identify potential problem areas.

Mechanisms for Minimizing Costs

Subcontracting can be a useful mechanism for minimizing the cost of research activities that require special skills not readily available from existing staff. Examples are as varied as laboratory testing, patient interviewing, and computer data entry. Qualified subcontractors are more than happy to provide estimates of the charge for their work. This process will require the researcher to specify what is involved. To estimate data entry charges, for example, the subcontractor would need to know at a minimum the number of records, the length of each, the type of data (strictly numeric versus character) and whether verification is desired (i.e., re-entry of data to identify and correct keypunch errors).

Research costs can be minimized also by using existing data collected for other purposes and by incorporating research tasks in the ongoing responsibilities of existing staff. These strategies have their limitations, however. First of all, existing data sources rarely include all needed information in the desired form. More importantly, the quality of the data is unknown. Clinical research has a low threshold for errors and omissions, and sources suitable for other purposes may be substandard from a research perspective. If use of existing data is contemplated, it is essential that a feasibility study be conducted to ascertain the quality of these data.

Another strategy to minimize research costs is to incorporate research tasks in the ongoing responsibilities of program personnel. If nonresearch personnel will be expected to perform study tasks in addition to their regular duties, however, special efforts must be made to assure both their understanding of the research protocol and their continued adherence to it. For example, suppose a study requires collection of specific information on household composition (number of persons in the household and age, sex and relationship of each) at each well child visit. Clinic staff could solicit the information at the time of registration. Alternatively, nursing staff could do so at the time height and weight are measured. In either instance, staff will not perform even a simple task such as this consistently unless they are taught how and why it is important to do so. Furthermore, unless these points are reinforced through periodic review and feedback on staff performance and study progress, consistency will fall off as competing job demands gain staff attention.

"Money is a good servant but a bad master" (*Bacon*). It is important that researchers do not fall into the trap of writing a grant to perform a study that they do not find especially interesting or for which they are not completely prepared just because money is available. Otherwise a lot of time and energy will be wasted preparing it; however, if they are lucky (or unlucky) enough to receive the grant, it might dampen or totally drown any interest in future studies.

Funding

Securing funding can be one of the most consuming and frustrating aspects of clinical research. The array of both public and private funding sources is complex. For many sources, research priorities change over time. The application process and eligibility requirements vary enormously by funding source. Finally, the time period from proposal submission to project funding (or notification of denial) often stretches to 1 year.

For the beginning researcher, the procedures for securing funding, particularly federal funding, may be imposing. Certainly, many first-time research projects are doable on modest, locally obtained funding coupled with a very generous input of time from the investigator and his or her colleagues; however, since few researchers can afford to continue with little or no funding forever, the focus of this section is relevant both for the novice researcher, and for those contemplating outside funding for the first time.

Competition for both public and private research support is keen. To illustrate, of the 1,290 research proposals submitted to the Center for Research for Mothers and Children (CRMC) of the National Institute of Child Health and Human Development (NICHD) in fiscal year 1985, only 283 were funded. Furthermore, it has been estimated that nearly four of five applications to private foundations are inappropriate or misdirected (Peterson 1985). To avoid this pitfall, to increase the efficiency of fundraising efforts and the likelihood of their success, the following common sense guidelines should be followed:

1. Become acquainted with the basic facts about public and private funding sources in general.
2. Define areas of research interest and identify sources of support with similar research interests and priorities.
3. Obtain detailed information on the funding history, eligibility requirements, and application procedures of identified sources of support.
4. Write a letter of intent, including the proposed funding necessary, to those organizations that seem most appropriate. For sources of support that respond with a request for a full proposal, prepare and submit one that complies with the source's specific instructions regarding format, content, length, number of copies, and application deadlines.

Funding Sources

This section provides background information on the types of support available for clinical research, the array of funding sources through which they are offered, strategies for identifying potential sources of support and general aspects of the application process.

The information presented here is intended only to serve as a starting point in defining the funding options open to the pediatric clinical researcher and the ways to explore and pursue those most appropriate to his or her interests. There are many published references on all aspects of research funding and, more recently, computer-based references as well. Some of these are included in the suggested readings in this chapter. Colleagues and professional organizations can provide invaluable information on funding opportunities. Most medical institutions engaged in research maintain an office of research administration with current reference materials on funding sources and trained staff eager to be of assistance. It would be wise to make full use of all these resources in the quest for support.

Research support takes many forms. Chief among them are the contract and the grant. Other types of support include cooperative arrangements, fellowships, and donations or gifts.

Contract

A contract is a legal agreement in which the funding source procures a specific service or product (i.e., the conduct of research to answer questions the funding source specifies via methods it also specifies). No change in study objective, scope or methods can be made prior to explicit funding agency approval.

Grant

This is the most common form of research support. It is less restrictive than a contract, and although the researcher must comply with technical and financial report requirements, autonomy is given in defining research goals and methods. Whereas contract support is limited to procurement of a specified service or product, the scope of grant support extends to basic research. Various sponsors including federal agencies, foundations, and corporations offer grant support.

The best known form of federal grant support is the research project grant, which provides funding for a discrete, specified project to be performed by the investigator in his or her area of interest and expertise. In addition to the research project grant, however, the federal government offers a wide variety of assistance mechanisms for support of research. For example, some agencies offer small grant support for pilot projects and feasibility studies of no longer than 1 year and with direct costs generally not in excess of $15,000.

Another support mechanism of particular interest to new researchers is the First Independent Research Support and Transition (FIRST) award, which is offered by many of the institutes including those responsible for most pediatric research funding. Details on FIRST award features, application procedures and participating National Institutes of Health (NIH) agencies are presented in the *NIH Guide to Grants and Contracts* (Vol. 15, No. 4, March 28, 1986).

Cooperative Agreement

The cooperative agreement is a relatively new form of federal support for a discrete, specified, circumscribed project to be performed by the researcher in an area representing his or her specific interests and competencies. It is used in lieu of a grant when substantial programmatic involvement is anticipated between the federal funding agency and the researcher during performance of the project.

Fellowship

A fellowship is an award to support advanced or continued education in a specified research area. Like grants, fellowships are offered by a variety of funding agencies in both the public and private sectors.

Donation/Gift

In general, these are funds provided to a medical institution without intended benefit to the donor. Unlike other sources of support, donors do not usually require detailed technical and financial reports, although progress report letters are an expected courtesy.

Public Funding Sources

Most pediatric research support comes from the federal government, notably the NIH. This section presents several key points of a recent examination of the growth and development of federally funded pediatric research (Stiehm 1985). Within NIH, two agencies provide the bulk of pediatric research funding: the Clinical Research Center (CRC) program of the Division of Research Resources and the NICHD. The CRC program supports 75 centers nationally, most of them at teaching hospitals. About one third of CRC funding is devoted to pediatric research; a similar proportion of the trainees in its clinical associate physician program have been pediatricians.

NICHD is the largest source of research support for pediatric departments, devoting about one sixth of its funds to pediatric research. Other institutes making significant contributions to pediatric research include the National Institutes of Allergy, Digestive and Metabolic Disease; the National Heart and Lung Institute; National Institute of Allergy, Immunology and Infectious Diseases; and the National Cancer Institute.

Federal research support to pediatric departments and individual children's hospitals totalled nearly $82 million in 1983. Most support is concentrated in a few large research-oriented institutions. To illustrate, 5 (4 percent) of the 120 departments nationwide received a total of 207 (36 percent) of the NIH pediatric research grants awarded in 1983, while the majority of departments (55 percent) received only 1 pediatric research grant or none at all.

It should be noted that state and local agencies, particularly health departments, occasionally have research funds to study problems specific to their jurisdiction. Certainly the availability of funding is far less than that offered directly at the federal level. Moreover, each local department has its own research priorities and application procedures. The most efficient way to learn what funding might be available is to contact the health department directly, particularly its research division and any other division related to the content area of interest (e.g., maternal and child health).

Private Funding Sources

Two other major sources of research support are private foundations and the drug industry. The drug industry tends to develop
working relationships with outside investigators on an individual
basis rather than soliciting research proposals from the research
community at large. For this reason, it will not be discussed as a
source of funding here, and the remainder of this section will focus
on private foundations.

Foundation grants totalled $4.36 billion in 1984, with 13 percent
allocated to research (Peterson 1985). While government funding
for research exceeds that of private foundations, the latter do offer
an excellent source of support for clinical researchers. This is
especially true for investigators whose research focus or approach
does not mesh well with the prevailing interests of governmental
funding agencies.

Not all private foundations award grants. For the purposes of this
discussion, a private foundation is defined as a nongovernmental,
nonprofit organization with funds and programs managed by its
own trustees or directors and established to maintain or aid the
common welfare by making grants to other nonprofit organizations. There are five basic types of private foundations: national,
special interest, corporate, family, and community.

National Foundations

National foundations are usually quite large and do not limit their
support to any geographic area. Examples include The Robert
Wood Johnson Foundation and the Rockefeller Foundation. In
general, foundations of this type prefer projects with implications at
least at the regional level and preferably at the national level.
Because of their size, national foundations can fund relatively large
projects and competition for their support is especially keen.

Special Interest Foundations

These are foundations and associations that focus exclusively on a
single field. Examples include the American Heart Association, the
March of Dimes, the American Cancer Society; and the many other
associations supporting research on a specific disease. Like national

foundations, special interest foundations usually do not limit their activities geographically.

Corporate Foundations

There are close to 300 foundations serving as the philanthropic arm of their founding corporations. These foundations tend to limit their funding to projects in keeping with the sponsoring corporation's business interests. Two corporate foundations with research interests in pediatrics are the Hasbro Children's Foundation and the Mattel Foundation.

Family Foundations

Family foundations comprise the largest number of private foundations. They vary enormously in size and area of interest. Most are small and fund projects related to the individual interests of family members. Grant awards also tend to be relatively small and are frequently limited to the locality in which the family resides or conducts business. Examples of family foundations interested in pediatrics and child welfare are the Charles H. Hood Foundation, the Laidlaw Foundation, and the Henry J. Kaiser Family Foundation.

Community Foundations

Community foundations are public charities that derive their funds from public support and direct their grants to the community they serve and for which they are named. There are approximately 250 community foundations nationwide. A local trust bank can provide information on the existence of a community foundation in its area.

Identifying Potential Sources of Support

As noted earlier, most federal research support is awarded in the form of grants and contracts. Proposals for grant funding may be either solicited or unsolicited; all proposals for contract funding are solicited. A solicited grant or contract proposal is one submitted in response to a formal Request for Applications (RFA) issued by a governmental agency that sponsors extramural research (e.g., the NICHD, and the Alcohol, Drug Abuse and Mental Health Administration or ADAMHA). An RFA is a statement of the agency's intent to fund research addressing a specific issue. The statement usually includes background information, the funding objectives, eligibility requirements, review criteria, application instructions, and the projected dates for funding availability.

In addition to funding solicited research proposals, most federal and private agencies earmark a portion of their extramural research budgets for unsolicited proposals to study issues within the agency's general areas of interest but not identified in problem-specific RFAs. Like RFAs, announcements of the availability of funding for unsolicited projects are published in the NIH Guide. Also published as announcements are statements on the availability of research support via mechanisms other than the traditional research project grant (e.g., FIRST awards).

Most agencies publish detailed summaries and progress reports of their recent extramural research as well as explicit narratives on upcoming research initiatives and priorities. Examples of recent NICHD publications in these areas include the 1985 *Progress Report of NICHD's Center for Research for Mothers and Children* (GPO 921-198), the agency's April 1986 *Special Report to Congress*, and its 1983 publication of *An Overview and Strategy for a Five-Year Research Plan* (U.S. GPO 1983 0-381-132/3207). The most efficient way to gather information on an agency's research priorities and the availability of funds for unsolicited proposals is by contacting the agency directly.

Within the private sector, most foundations publish annual reports that provide information on what they fund. Foundation annual reports are often kept on file as references in an institution's central research administration office. In addition, copies can be obtained by writing directly to the foundation.

Several general references on both public and private funding sources are available to the researcher. Among these are the registers and directories listed at the end of this chapter. Such references are usually available in public, medical, and other educational institution libraries. Foundation entries are categorized and indexed by several characteristics, including field of interest and geographic area of awards. By using the indexes, it is a simple (though time-consuming) process to identify foundations with a common research interest.

In addition to published registers and directories, computer data bases of funding sources are now available. Among these are the Sponsored Programs Information Network (SPIN) developed by the State University of New York and the Illinois Researcher Information System (IRIS) of the University of Illinois at Urbana. These computerized online telecommunications networks are designed to provide up-to-date complete information on research support available in both the private and public sectors. Data system personnel gather and update funding information on a continuing basis from funding references published periodically and from annual reports of private sponsors. As with published directories, each funding source is categorized and indexed by keyword codes referring to its areas of interest. By selecting one or a combination of keyword codes, the researcher can obtain an annotated printout of all funding sources sharing the same area of interest.

Both published and computer-based directories contain a wealth of useful information about each funding source listed. This includes name, address, telephone number, purpose and activities, number of grants awarded annually, size of awards (minimum, maximum, usual), eligibility requirements, how to apply (what to submit, when, and to whom), application review and award schedule, and whom to contact for additional information. Table 6.2 provides a brief annotated bibliography of related references for sources of research support.

Applying for Research Support

In its simplest form, the proposal itself is a well-organized presentation of evidence constituting a logical and compelling argument in support of the research. The proposal begins with a statement of research aims, including the specific research questions to be answered and hypotheses to be tested. Following this is an examination of the background of the study, including evaluation of existing knowledge both to demonstrate the importance of the proposed research and to provide the rationale for study hypotheses.

TABLE 6.2.   Annotated Bibliography of Selected References
for Sources of Research Support

Annual Register of Grant Support. 20th ed. Petersen, L., ed. Wilmette: National
Register Publishing Company, 1986.

Includes both public and private granting sources. Organized by disciplines. Indexed according to subject, geographic locations, organizations, and personnel.

Catalog of Federal Domestic Assistance. United States Office of Economic Opportunity. Washington, DC: The Office of Management and Budget.

Compiled and published annually by the Federal Office of Management and
Budget, the catalog provides the user with access to all assistance and benefit
programs of federal departments and agencies, including loans, subsidies and
technical assistance programs. Program information is cross-referenced by
agency, functional classification, subject, eligibility requirements, popular name,
authorizing legislation, and federal circular requirements.

Commerce Business Daily. United States Department of Commerce: Chicago.

Daily list of U.S. government procurement invitations, contract awards, subcontracting leads, sales of surplus property and foreign business opportunities.

Federal Register. United States Government Printing Office, The Office of the
Federal Register.

Publicizes regulations and legal notices issued by federal agencies. Includes announcements of grant availability and proposed and final issuances of administrative regulations.

The Foundation Directory. 10th ed. Renz, L., ed. New York: The Foundation
Center, 1985.

Describes nonfederal, nonprofit foundations with assets in excess of $1 million
or that make grants totaling $500,000 or more annually.

The Foundation Grant Index. 15th ed. Garonzic, E., ed. New York: The Foundation Center, 1986.

Lists foundation grants of $5000 or more. Foundations are listed alphabetically
and by state. Other indexes include recipient, subject categories, and keywords/
phrases referring to grant description and type of recipient organization. Published yearly.

NIH Guide to Grants and Contracts United States Department of Health and
Human Service, National Institutes of Health. Bethesda.

Weekly publication of Requests for Applications (RFAs) for solicited research
project grants, announcements of the availability of funding via other mechanisms, including description of funding objectives, eligibility requirements, and
instructions on how to obtain additional information. Entries are arranged by
institute.

TABLE 6.2. (continued)

National Science Foundation Guide to Programs

An annually updated summary by area of NSF basic research funding opportunities and points of contact.

Research Awards Index. vol. I and II. United States Department of Health and Human Services, Public Health Service, National Institutes of Health, Division of Research Grants, Washington, DC: United States Government Printing Office.

Annual Public Health Service publication of information on health research currently conducted by nonfederal institutions and supported by NIH, ADAMHA, FDA, and HRA. Useful in identifying recent research activities in specific areas.

Having established the need for the proposed research and its theoretical soundness, the researcher should then provide evidence of competence to carry it out, as indicated by a review of past experience in preliminary studies related to the research area and/or using the proposed methodology. The methods section follows, and at a minimum it defines the study population and sample, the study design, the sources, measurement, and quality (i.e., validity and reliability) of the data to be collected, data collection procedures, the scheduling of steps in the research process, and the analytic plan. The proposal concludes with a description of the interpretation and implications of study findings and proposed methods for their dissemination.

Although some federal research support programs have their own application forms and procedures, most use Form PHS 398, the Application for Public Health Service Grant. This form or any other required by an agency may be obtained directly from the agency offering research support. Form PHS 398 contains all needed application materials and complete instructions for preparing the grant proposal, including the budget, research plan, and assurance of the protection of human subjects.

The most common error in proposal preparation is failure to follow the application instructions compulsively. Reviewers are responsible for reading and evaluating an enormous amount of material in a short period of time. Their work is minimized to the extent that the proposals they read are uniform in format. Departures from the requested format make it difficult for the reviewers to find key information and increase the likelihood that proposal elements will be misunderstood or missed entirely. This, in turn, jeopardizes a favorable funding decision.

Basically, there are three overlapping federal grant application review and award cycles per year, with application receipt dates of February 1, June 1, and October 1, as shown in Table 6.3. It should be noted that the minimum time from proposal submission to project starting date for new grants is 9 months. Quite often, notification of funding decisions is not made until within 1 month of project startup. These characteristics of the application and funding schedule underscore the importance of long-term planning, particularly the development of alternatives in the event that funding is denied.

Most private foundations suggest that first contact be made via a letter of intent in which the researcher *briefly* describes himself or herself and the proposed project. The foundation can then determine whether the proposed research should be considered for funding. In this way, the foundation does not waste time reviewing full proposals for projects that are inappropriate for its funding objectives. More important for the researcher, no effort is misspent preparing a detailed proposal that has no chance of funding.

Each foundation has its own requirements regarding proposal content and format, which should be followed to the letter. Of particular importance is the project abstract or summary, which should be a clear, concise description of the project. It is often used by reviewers as a screen to determine which proposals are reviewed in their entirety.

Ethical Standards for Research Involving Human Subjects

The Public Health Service Act calls for protection of the rights of human research subjects through informed consent. Federal regulations in this regard are documented in Title 45, Part 46 of the *Code of Federal Regulations of the Department of Health and Human Services* (DHHS). The regulations apply to all research funded by

TABLE 6.3. Public Health Service Research Application Review
and Award Schedule

Receipt Dates*	Initial Review Group Dates	National Advisory Council/Board Dates	Earliest Possible Beginning Dates
Feb 1	June	Sept/Oct	Dec 1
June 1	Oct/Nov	Jan/Feb	April 1
Oct 1	Feb/March	May/June	July 1

*For most new research grant applications. Dates 1 month later are used for all competing continuation and supplemental applications as well as special applications such as FIRST awards.

the DHHS and/or falling within the purview of the Food and Drug Administration. At the institutional level, policy regarding the protection of human rights is based on federal requirements but usually extends beyond them.

The Scope of Federal Regulations

The DHHS regulations for the protection of human subjects define a human subject as a "living individual about whom an investigator (whether professional or student) conducting research obtains (1) data through intervention or interaction with the individual, or (2) identifiable private information." The regulations apply to research involving the use of human organs, tissues, and body fluids from individually identifiable human subjects and to do research involving recording information from individually identifiable human subjects. Children and prisoners are afforded special protections under the regulations. There are also additional protections pertaining to research involving fetuses, pregnant women, and human invitro fertilization. Finally, the intent of DHHS regulations extends to human subject research limited to self-experimentation by the investigator and staff. Research limited to one or more of the following five activities is exempt from coverage by the DHHS regulations:

1. Research conducted in established or commonly accepted educational settings involving normal educational practices, such as

research on regular and special education instructional strategies, or research on the effectiveness of or the comparison among instructional techniques, curriculums, or classroom management methods.

2. Research involving the use of educational tests (cognitive, diagnostic, aptitude, achievement), if information taken from these sources is recorded in such a manner that subjects cannot be identified directly or through identifiers linked to the subjects.

3. Research involving survey or interview procedures and/or observation (including observation by participants) of public behavior, except where all of the following conditions exist: (a) responses/observations are recorded in such a manner that the human subjects can be identified directly or through identifiers linked to the subjects; (b) the subject's responses/observed behavior, if they became known outside the research, could reasonably place the subject at risk of criminal or civil liability or be damaging to the subject's financial standing or employability; and (c) the research deals with sensitive aspects of the subject's own behavior, such as illegal conduct, drug use, sexual behavior, or use of alcohol. All research involving survey or interview procedures is exempt, without exception, when the respondents are elected or appointed public officials or candidated for public office.

4. Research involving the collection or study of existing data, documents, records, pathological specimens, or diagnostic specimens, if these sources are publicly available or if the information is recorded by the investigator in such a manner that subject cannot be identified directly or through identifiers linked to the subjects.

5. Research involving the observation of public behavior except when (a) observations are recorded in such a way that the human subjects can be identified, (b) the recorded observations, if they become known outside the research, could reasonably place the subject at risk of criminal or civil liability or be damaging to the subject's financial standing or employability, and (c) the research deals with sensitive aspects of the subject's behavior, e.g., illegal conduct, drug use, sexual behavior, alcohol use.

Institutional Framework for Assuring Protection of Rights

The DHHS requires each institution engaged in research involving human subjects to file an Assurance of Compliance with the Office for Protection from Research Risks, specifying the institution's research review policy and procedures. Central to this is the institution's establishment of a standing Institutional Review Board (IRB) with responsibility for review and approval of all the institution's research projects and activities subject to protection of the rights of human subjects under federal law.

While the DHHS regulations apply primarily to federally funded research, institutional policy on human subjects often extends beyond this to privately funded or nonfunded research as well. For example, a hospital might require IRB approval of *any* research involving its patients or their records, regardless of funding source or exempt status under federal regulations. In addition, institutional policy might require IRB approval or all human subject research conducted by its members, regardless of the source of the subjects. To illustrate, a medical school might require its faculty to obtain IRB approval for all their research projects, even those conducted in other institutions or in the field.

Large scale or collaborative studies may involve multiple sites. Some institutions have developed cooperative agreements to minimize duplicative effort for studies where more than one IRB might have jurisdiction. In studies with multiple sites, the principal investigator should consult the IRB of the institution of her primary affiliation to determine whether review by other IRBs will be required.

In summary, within each institution the IRB has ultimate responsibility for safeguarding the rights of human subjects in research. Since IRB policies and procedures vary by institution, the best advice is to consult the IRB while in the early stages of research design. The IRB can provide the investigator with copies of the DHHS and Food and Drug Administration regulations [45 CFR 46 and Federal Register 46 (17):8942–80, January 27, 1981] and will determine whether the proposed research requires or is exempt from its review and approval. Where review is required, the IRB will determine whether proposed study procedures are sufficient to safeguard the rights of human subjects. Finally, where approval is denied, the IRB will outline what changes in study protocol are needed.

General Requirements for Informed Consent

Subject consent to participate in a study must be informed; that is, it must be based on a clear understanding of the research as it applies to participants. Investigators are required to obtain informed consent in writing, with some exceptions (e.g., telephone surveys and instances where the only document linking research and identifying information would be the signed statement). This is accomplished by preparing an informed consent statement to be read and signed by the subjects as a prerequisite to participation.

Parental consent is required in studies involving children. The nature of study procedures as well as the age of the child should be considered in assessing whether and how to obtain the child's assent. For young children, the investigator might explain the study orally at an appropriate level. Older children and adolescents can be furnished with their own simply worded assent statement.

The informed consent statement should be written in clear, concise language. Where study subgroups are exposed to different procedures, separate group-specific consent forms should be composed to simplify content.

The DHHS regulations define "basic elements" of informed consent (i.e., aspects of the research for which information must be provided to each subject). First, the statement must describe the purpose of the study and the reasons the subject qualifies for participation. The statement must also include a simple explanation for the study design, procedures involving the subject, and the methods used to determine assignment of treatment groups. Each aspect of participation should be specified (e.g., number, timing, general content and length of interviews, required clinic visits, laboratory tests) and each activity conducted solely for research purposes must be identified as such.

The informed consent statement must also describe both potential risks (including discomfort) and benefits to subjects. The severity and likelihood of major risks in particular must be specified. The consent statement must also explain whether any compensation and/or medical treatments are available if injury occurs as a result of study participation and either describe what is available or explain where additional information may be obtained.

Often, subjects are not expected to benefit directly from study participation. If this is so, it must be stated. On the other hand, if potential benefits for science, other patients or the general public are expected, these should be noted in the consent statement. Finally, if subjects are to be remunerated for participation, the informed consent statement should indicate the amount.

Subjects must be appraised of the alternative to study participation. In clinical studies, this usually means disclosure of procedures or courses of treatment, if any, that might be advantageous to the subject but that are not offered as a part of study participation.

The informed consent statement must make the voluntary nature of participation clear to the subject, including his or her right to withdraw from the study at any time. The statement must explain that refusal to participate or to continue in the study will involve no penalty or less of benefits to which the subject is otherwise entitled.

The extent to which the confidentiality of study records will be maintained should be noted. Finally, the statement must indicate whom the subject should contact for questions about the study or research subjects' rights or in the event of a research-related injury or complaint.

In addition to the required elements of informed consent, there are additional elements that are appropriate in particular circumstances. Among these are statements regarding (1) the possibility of unforeseeable risks to the subject; (2) circumstances under which the investigator may terminate the subject's participation; (3) additional costs to the subject that might result from study; (4) the investigator's intent to notify subjects of new findings that might affect the subject's willingness to continue study participation; and (5) the approximate number of study subjects.

Federal regulations empower the IRB to approve deviations from the standard elements of informed consent. Individual IRBs may elect to require elements in addition to those mandated by DHHS. Again, the investigator's best strategy is to consult the institution's review board early in the study's planning stages to determine what elements of informed consent will require and, in studies involving children, whether and what type of assent procedures should be used.

Collaboration

As noted earlier, the limitations imposed by the modest budgets of many research efforts are balanced by the generous amount of effort donated by the investigator and his or her colleagues. While more elaborate studies might enjoy the benefits of substantial funding, the importance of collaboration is not diminished. Colleagues might or might not be paid for their efforts, and the reasons for collaboration might be different (e.g., the need for multiple study sites versus the importance of a multidisciplinary approach), but the key issue of collaboration is applicable in both large and small projects. The most important consideration in developing collaborative arrangements is to set the ground rules at the onset. This means establishing the role of each collaborator and the interrelationships involved. It also means defining the anticipated level of effort of each researcher throughout the course of the study. Finally, it means agreeing beforehand on the plans for dissemination of study findings and authorship.

It is unfortunate how frequently investigators fail to address these issues directly. The likelihood of misunderstanding is minimized if the details of collaboration are discussed fully and summarized in writing. In this way, collaborator consent to participation in the study, like that of the study subjects, is informed. In short, explicit collaborative agreements increase both the probability of successful study completion and the desirability of subsequent collaborative efforts.

Suggested Readings

Petersen, L. ed. *The Annual Register of Grant Support: a directory of funding sources.* Wilmette: National Register Publishing Company, 1985.

Stiehm, E. R. "Growth and Development of Pediatric Research." *Pediatr Res* 19: (1985) 593–98.

7

How to Read a Publication

WILLIAM FELDMAN

How to Read a Medical Journal Article

For most doctors reading the literature is the preferred form of
continuing medical education, ranking higher than attending
rounds, listening to audiotapes, and attending national or interna-
tional conferences. Although there is no proof that physicians who
regularly read journal articles provide better care to their patients
than those who do not, intuitively one feels that reading is a good
thing. Most of us engaged in academic medicine read a lot and
encourage our trainees, by our own example and by pushing and
prodding, to do likewise. We therefore have an obligation to ensure
that we and those we teach know how to read a journal article.

Everybody who succeeded in medical school knows how to read
a journal—don't they? Not necessarily. In fact most medical education at the student and resident level is not geared to a proper
critical appraisal of the literature. Critical appraisal means that the
reader has the appropriate understanding of clinical research methodologies, knows the criteria by which to evaluate the quality of the
evidence presented by the author, and can judge whether to use the
results of the study in practice. It is important to remember that
statistical significance is not the same as clinical significance. Clini-

cal journal articles can be classified as providing information primarily in one of five categories: etiology, diagnosis, prognosis, therapy, or screening. The following discussion is based on those categories of publication.

How to Read an Article on Etiology or Causation of Disease

Reading an article critically involves the same knowledge base as performing the study that is reported in the article.

The best proof that something causes a disease in a subject—for example *Escherichia coli* 0157:H7 causing the hemolytic-uremic syndrome—would be an experiment in which the investigator would randomly allocate one group of subjects to ingest *E. coli* 0157:H7 and another group to ingest another serotype. The investigator would then determine the proportion of subjects in each group who developed hemolytic-uremic syndrome. This type of research (i.e., the randomized control trial), while scientifically ideal, is usually morally unacceptable, and is not commonly performed to determine etiology.

The type of study that is next in order of scientific soundness in determining etiology is the cohort study. Suppose several hundred campers and counsellors in a summer camp are unintentionally exposed to drinking water or food contaminated with *E. coli* 0157:H7. The investigator could determine how many were infected with the organism and how many were not, and follow-up both groups to determine the proportion of those infected and not infected who developed the disease. If there were a statistically significant increase in disease in the infected group, it could be assumed that there is a possible causal relationship between this serotype and the disease.

Next in order of credibility of evidence is the case–control study. In this type of study the investigator would identify patients with hemolytic-uremic syndrome and look for *E. coli* 0157:H7 in them as well as in healthy control subjects. A statistically significant increase in *E. coli* 0157:H7 in the cases when compared with the controls would suggest that there might be a causal relationship.

The reader will note that in the cohort study, "a possible causal relationship" was implied, and in the case–control study the results "would suggest that there might be a causal relationship." The reason for hedging about causality in both of these types of studies is that unless the investigator is in complete control of the study, as would occur in an experiment, there may be confounding variables that could mask the true cause. In the cohort example, it may be that the subjects infected with *E. coli* 0157:H7 also ate more of some other food or drank more of the water that contained another, as yet unidentified, organism or toxin that was the true cause of the illness. In the case–control example, the healthy controls may have had less *E. coli* 0157:H7 because they were healthier to begin with (i.e., perhaps certain host factors constitute the real cause of hemolytic-uremic syndrome and the cases had more *E. coli* 0157:H7 not because that serotype caused the disease but because subjects genetically predisposed to hemolytic-uremic syndrome may respond in this manner to a variety of agents). In this example the *E. coli* 0157:H7 may be a marker but not the cause of disease.

The least convincing type of investigation is the case series. An example of this is a recent report in which 14 children with hemolytic-uremic syndrome were studied. Seven of these children had *E. coli* 0157:H7 isolated and, therefore, causality was implied. The major problem with this study is that the authors did not describe the incidence of isolates of *E. coli* 0157:H7 in children who did not have hemolytic-uremic syndrome. Instead, they stated that standard microbiologic laboratory practice does not regularly include detailed characterization of *E. coli*. It is possible that 50 percent of the children with hemolytic-uremic syndrome had *E. coli* 0157:H7 because the authors were looking for it. Since most children with diarrhea do not have stool cultures, and since those that do, rarely have serotyping performed, it is possible that *E. coli* 0157:H7 is more prevalent than was previously thought and may not be causally related to the hemolytic-uremic syndrome.

In summary, the best evidence about causation comes from randomized controlled trials. Since these are not always ethically feasible, the more common form of evidence available is the result of a cohort study. Next in credibility is the case–control study. The closer the subjects who are exposed to the putative cause are in relation to those nonexposed—with regard to important possible confounding factors such as age, sex, social class—and risk of exposure to other potential causes, the more credible is the study. Case series, however, can also provide important information especially as clues for causation that can then be better tested by cohort, case control, or even randomized controlled trials.

How to Read a Journal Article on Diagnosis

When an article describes a diagnostic approach, the careful reader should look for some methodologic features of the study that would help to determine how useful the test would be in practice. First, were the subjects who were studied similar to those the reader is likely to encounter in practice? The most important bias to look for is the *referral bias*. Most articles describing a diagnostic approach involve subspecialists using subjects from university centers, where the cases studied are often the most difficult. Years ago, the investigation of hypertension in children included costly and fairly risky tests such as renal arteriograms and renal vein renin assays. The original studies showing a fairly high yield, (i.e., 78 percent), were from those referral centers managing the toughest cases; in primary care only 5 percent of cases of hypertension are secondary. Most physicians caring for children with hypertension have now been advised to try simpler approaches such as salt restriction, weight reduction, and so on before referring. Many hypertensive children and adolescents will improve on this regime, especially the large number with a family history of essential hypertension. If these children had been referred and studied, the results showing a high number of cases of renovascular hypertension would not have been so dramatic and the true, low prevalence of this condition would have been recognized.

Second, how good is the diagnostic test when compared with a gold standard of diagnosis? For example, in considering whether ultrasound of the kidneys, ureters and bladder can replace the intravenous pyelogram (IVP) in assessing patients with urinary tract infections, it is important that the study describe a group of subjects with and without pyelographic changes whose ultrasounds were read blindly by ultrasonographers in an attempt to see how closely the ultrasound approached the gold standard IVP.

Third, how objective and accurate is the test? For example, if the investigator showed the same ultrasounds to the same observer at two separate points in time, how often would the previous interpretation be questioned (intra-observer reliability)? If they were shown to two separate observers, how often would they agree (inter-observer reliability)? If ultrasounds were performed on the same subject 1 day after the original one, how much alike would they be (reproducibility)?

Fourth, was the term *abnormal* defined in a sensible manner? For example, many laboratory-oriented physicians define an abnormal result as one that is greater than two standard deviations from the mean. This definition, while statistically abnormal, has nothing to do with sickness or health. If being two standard deviations off the mean signified illness, all persons with leukocyte counts less than $4,500/mm^3$ would be ill. A better definition of abnormal would be a finding that has been shown to lead to improved health in those with the finding who are treated when compared with those with the finding who are not treated. The patient has to be better off for having had the test performed and the diagnosis made than if they were not.

In summary, in reading an article on diagnosis, the reader must be sure that the diagnostic approach or tests used are on subjects similar to his or her own patients, and that the test is as good as the gold standard, and has features of safety or cost that make it preferable. In addition, the test should be objective and usable by different persons to get the same results. Abnormal findings should be defined not in statistical terms but as results that, when followed up and treated, led to more good than harm.

How to Read an Article on Prognosis

The first point to consider in reviewing an article on prognosis is whether or not an inception cohort was assembled. This means that all the subjects followed should have come under observation either before they were symptomatic or at a uniformly early point in the course of the disease. For example, in order to know what to tell parents of a child who has just suffered a first simple febrile seizure, it is important to review long-term follow-up studies of children who were very similar to this patient. We know from birth cohort studies that the child with no underlying neurologic dysfunction who has a short-lived generalized febrile seizure with no focal findings has an excellent prognosis both with regard to afebrile seizures and normal mental development. On the other hand, if the study includes a different population of subjects who have seizures with fever, including those who are neurologically or developmentally abnormal to start with, or who have focal seizures, the prognosis is not as good.

Next, the referral pattern must be described. If the study follows a group of subjects with febrile seizures from a neurology clinic, they may have more complicated disease, and therefore, a different prognosis than subjects followed in office practice with a more representative disease severity.

Third, was complete follow-up achieved? Even if one starts with a proper cohort of subjects who resemble those in your practice, if even a few subjects missed follow-up, the interpretation may be difficult. For example, the prognosis of certain types of seizures would be falsely optimistic if all those who subsequently died of status epilepticus were not alive and therefore were not followed up. This is an unlikely scenario, but one that helps to make the point.

Fourth, in determining the final status (healthy versus unhealthy) of those who constituted the inception cohort, were the criteria of healthy versus unhealthy explicit and objective, and were those who rated them blind to the subject's original condition? For example, in deciding whether children who had previously had febrile seizure were or were not developmentally normal at the conclusion of the study, were objective measures of development used? Similarly, were those who were administering the developmental tests aware of the underlying neurological status of the child? If so, their testing and interpretation may have been biased.

In summary, in reading an article on prognosis the reader must look for the presence of an inception cohort, and ensure that the subjects who were followed up were similar to those in his or her practice. All subjects should be accounted for at the end of the study, and the means used to ascertain the health status of the cohort members at the conclusion of the study should be explicit and objective.

How to Read an Article on Therapy

It is important that the reader avoid wasting time reading articles on therapy that are not the result of randomized trials, and hopefully double-blind, randomized trials. If this standard had been applied, there would be many more persons with intact tonsils and foreskins, and fewer manufacturers of kaolin and pectin.

First randomization has to be truly random (i.e., once informed consent has been given, every patient must have an equal probability of receiving one of the regimens being studied). If chart numbers or days of the week are used to designate to which group the subject is assigned, it is possible to have unconscious bias. For example, in an actual study comparing sponging and antipyretics with antipyretics alone to reduce fever, the nurses knew to which group the subject would be assigned by looking at the chart number. It is possible that some subjects were not approached to be in the study because one or more of the nurses may have had a bias in favor of sponging. Thus it is possible that only those subjects who were felt to be well enough to be in the study were enrolled, and those who were felt to need sponging were not. If the nurse knew the subjects would be in the sponging group they might be approached. If the nurse knew the subjects were to be in the other group, they may not have been approached. To demonstrate that the randomization was successful, a table should be made to show that both the study and control groups were similar in age, sex, race, social class, and disease severity before therapy was instituted.

Second, all clinically relevant outcomes should be reported. For example, it is clear that the recurrence rate of febrile seizures can be reduced by giving prophylactic phenobarbital, but in this case, the treatment may be worse than the disease. The resultant behavioral and cognitive effects of the drug may have more deleterious effects than would recurrent febrile seizures.

Third, as mentioned previously in the sections on diagnosis and prognosis, the researcher must be sure that the subjects described in the study are similar to those he or she would be treating. For example, an excellent prospective double-blind study showing methotrexate to be valuable in treating rheumatoid arthritis should not lead the investigator to jump on a methotrexate bandwagon before giving acetylsalicylic acid a good trial. The majority of patients with rheumatoid arthritis seen in primary care do very well with simple, less toxic drugs. The subjects treated with immunosuppressive therapy were studied because they were different from the type of patient likely to be seen in primary care in that they did not respond to usual treatment.

Fourth, were clinical and statistical significance both assessed? For example, treating iron deficiency without anemia has been shown to increase the intelligence quotient of infants by a few points, which proved to be statistically significant. But how important clinically are several I.Q. points? A physician must not be led into using a treatment because of improvements in statistics: the improvement must be clinically important for patients. In addition, in studies that show no difference statistically between the new treatment and the traditional one or placebo, it is important that the authors describe the "power" of the study. This means that the sample size studied has to be large enough for the author to be 80 or 90 percent certain that a clinically significant difference between the two groups was not missed.

Finally, as in the section on prognosis, were all the subjects who entered the trial accounted for at the conclusion? For example, it had been clear for some time that clofibrate could lower serum cholesterol levels. When a randomized controlled trial was finally done some years later, the results were confirmed; namely, that cholesterol was lower among *survivors* in the clofibrate group. Yet the mortality rate in the clofibrate group was 17 percent higher than that of the placebo group. It was only because the authors accounted for all the subjects who entered the trial that this significantly excess mortality associated with clofibrate was discovered.

In summary, the best articles on therapy are those in which proper randomization has occurred and the patient and physician are both unaware of which treatment is being given. All clinically relevant outcomes, including side effects and mortality, should be reported. The patients studied should be similar to those in the researcher's practice. Both clinical and statistical significance should be dealt with, and, for studies where there is no difference between groups, the sample size should be large enough to be sure no clinically significant difference has been missed. Finally, all the patients who entered the study should be accounted for at the conclusion of the study.

How to Read an Article on Screening

Screening is an organized attempt to detect among apparently healthy persons in the community disorders or risk factors of which they are unaware.

The following are useful guidelines to be used in reviewing an article that recommends that a screening program be shown to be effective in a randomized controlled trial? As discussed in the section on therapy, the best way to be sure that screening does more good than harm is to have evidence that the group of subjects randomly allocated to a screening program are better off than the control group not screened. Surprisingly, most screening programs have not been tested by this criterion.

In one study, children randomly allocated to have preschool developmental assessment were compared 3 years later to children who were screened but whose results were kept hidden, and to a third group of children who were not screened. No differences were found between those who had a positive screen where the results were made known and interventions begun, and those who had a positive screen where the results were not divulged. However, the parents of positive screenees who were made aware of the results were significantly more worried than were the parents who were not told. In other words, the labeled children who had intervention did no better academically or in developmental tests, but their parents suffered more. Thus, a widely employed practice of preschool developmental screening, when finally put to the test of a randomized controlled trial, was shown not only to do no good, but in addition was shown, by the labeling effect, to do harm.

Second, if an effectiveness trial with a positive result has not been carried out, has it at least been shown that early diagnosis really makes a difference? For phenylketonuria and hypothyroidism screening in the newborn period, this clearly seems to be the case. In other words, treatment of those two conditions, before evidence of developmental delay is manifested, is usually associated with a favorable outcome because there are efficacious treatments when these are employed before irreversible brain damage has occurred. Can the same be said for scoliosis screening? Probably not, because most mild curves do not progress with or without treatment. In addition, significant curves needing bracing can usually be identified by a careful physician in the office employing a technique called *case finding*.

Case finding is defined as looking for a condition, during an office visit, that is different from the one for which the patient came to see the physician. Thus if an 11- or 12-year-old girl comes to see the physician for another reason, it is wise to look briefly at the spine, knowing these girls are most at risk of mild scoliosis. Mass screening for scoliosis produces so many false positives and so much anxiety that many communities no longer employ this practice.

Third, in the absence of controlled screening trials, does the burden of suffering warrant a screening program? In the case of phenylketonuria and hypothyroidism the answer is yes. In the case of scoliosis screening, the answer is probably no.

Similarly, if and when a good screening test for cystic fibrosis in the newborn period becomes available, should it be done? It can be argued that it should be done only if there is evidence that those children whose diagnosis is delayed by several months or years suffer because of the delay. It is possible that mass screening for cystic fibrosis will uncover children with positive tests who will never have symptoms, or if so, not until late adulthood. To label these children and start them on a cystic fibrosis regime might produce a burden of suffering even greater than that induced by the delay in diagnosis until symptoms developed.

Fourth, does a good screening test exist? Are the reported false-positive and false-negative rates sufficiently low? Using a less than good screening test in a study would automatically negate any findings.

Fifth, does the program reach those who would benefit from it? For example, mammography of women who had no access because of financial constraints to diagnostic and therapeutic intervention would not necessarily be helpful.

Finally, will those who test positive on the screen comply with subsequent advice and intervention? Will patients go to the appropriate physicians for confirmation of their diagnosis? Finally, will they comply with the necessary intervention (i.e., a special diet for hypercholesterolemia)?

In summary, in reading to learn about new screening programs, randomized screening effectiveness trials should be sought. In the absence of controlled trials the physician must be sure that the treatment given early helps those who take it, that the burden of suffering borne by a delayed diagnosis is greater than that of labeling, that there is a good test and a good follow-up treatment program that can reach those who would benefit, and that the subsequent advice and treatment is such that positive screenees are likely to comply.

In the absence of the articles' author having addressed these issues, it is difficult to accept positive recommendations on screening. Some guidelines have been provided in this chapter to assist the reader of a clinical journal article. The reader is referred to the publications listed in the references for further discussion.

Suggested Readings

Department of Clinical Epidemiology and Biostatistics. McMaster University, Hamilton, Ontario. "How to Read Clinical Journals: II To learn about a diagnostic Test." *Can Med Assoc J* 124 (1981): 703.

Department of Clinical Epidemiology and Biostatistics. McMaster University, Hamilton, Ontario. "How to Read Clinical Journals: III To Learn the Clinical Course and Prognosis of Disease." *Can Med Assoc J* 124 (1981): 869.

Sackett, D. L.; Haynes, R. B.; and Tugwell, P. *Clinical Epidemiology: A Basic Science for Clin Med*, Boston, Toronto: Little, Brown and Company, 1985.

8

Annotated Bibliography

JOHN PASCOE AND REBECCA HENRY

Critical Appraisal of the Medical Literature

Original Research

Gehlbach, S. H. *Interpreting the Medical Literature: A Clinician's Guide.* Lexington, Massachusetts: D.C. Heath and Company, 1982.

> This book provides the reader with a very logical and readable approach to understanding research literature for the primary care physician. Numerous examples from clinical research are included making it easier to understand some of the abstract concepts typically found in research books. The organization of the book parallels the sequence of a research article giving the readers the necessary tools to evaluate the primary components of a research study. The chapters on interpreting statistical significance, predictive values, and risk are particularly helpful for individuals who appreciate practical examples of these concepts.

Riegelman, R. K. *Studying a Study and Testing a Test: How to Read the Medical Literature.* Boston: Little, Brown and Company, 1981.

> The aim of this book is to provide a step-by-step approach to clinical review of the medical literature. Assuming no prior training

in statistics or epidemiology, the author presents four self-contained units that explain how to evaluate studies, tests, rates, and statistics found in journal articles. The four units are: Studying a study, testing a test; rating a rate, and selecting a statistic. The book is easy to read and includes very useful flaw-catching exercises.

Sackett, David L.; Haynes, R. Brian; and Tugwell, Peter. *Clinical Epidemiology: A Basic Science for Clinical Medicine.* Boston: Little, Brown and Company, 1985.

Part III of this book is titled, "Keeping Up to Date." In it, the authors provide a helpful service to the practicing physician by describing a procedure for reviewing and evaluating one's own clinical performance. Also, in this section, there are chapters titled: How to Use a Library; How to Read a Clinical Journal; Creating Your Own Library; and Getting The Most From Continuing Education. The chapter on reading a clinical journal is a good summary of the guides that have appeared in the *Canadian Medical Association Journal* over the past years.

Reviewing and Integrating Research

Cooper, H. M. *The Integrative Research Review: A Systemic Approach.* Beverly Hills: Sage Publications, 1984.

This short book is an excellent introduction for how to conduct a systemic research review. The author provides many examples, figures, and checklists that are practical and easy to follow. Five stages for conducting a research review are examined in detail. They include: problem formation; data collection; data evaluating; analysis and interpreting; and presentation. The chapter on data evaluation is a particularly important one. The author presents a detailed description of the "quantitative revolution" in research reviews that replaces the traditional approach with a set of statistical techniques that assist the reviewer in drawing comparisons and conclusions about strengths of relationship and effect size from multiple independent studies.

Light, R. J., and Pillemer, D. B. *Summing Up: The Science of Reviewing Research.* Cambridge: Harvard University Press, 1985.

Prior to any study the researcher must undertake a review of previous research. This book offers six chapters that focus on basic steps in conducting a research review. A framework is presented that helps the first-timer organize the literature and synthesize the sometimes contradictory results. Examples are provided and a 10-question checklist for evaluating other research reviews. Very practical for beginning and experienced researchers. The chapter titles include: Organizing a Reviewing Strategy; Quantitate Procedures; Numbers and Narrative; What We have Learned; and Checklist for Evaluating Reviews. The authors, (like Cooper) also propose a quantitative method for comparing multiple studies. These statistical procedures allow the reviewer to make summary statements about the data sets from different studies. Some statistical background is assumed.

Research Methodology and Management

Alreck, P. L., and Settle, R. B. *The Survey Research Handbook*. Homewood, Illinois: Irwin Press, 1985.

As the name implies, this is a handbook that will guide a new researcher through the fundamentals of survey methodology. In addition to the usual topics in survey research, this book also includes an extensive chapter on scaling techniques that will be helpful to anyone constructing items for the first time. The chapter on statistical analysis and interpreting the results is more comprehensive than usually found in this type of book.

Daniels, S. R.; Greenberg, R. S.; and Ibrahim, M. A. "Etiologic Research in Pediatric Epidemiology." *J Pediatr* 102 (1983): 494–504.

The controversy over the cause of Reye Syndrome may have encouraged the authors to write this careful summary of the major elements of etiologic research. Topics discussed include the observational approach, risk assessment, and the classification of study designs.

Feinstein, A. R. *Clinical Epidemiology: The Architecture of Clinical Research*. Philadelphia: W. B. Saunders, 1985.

This 800-page tome reflects Professor Feinstein's "activities at the Yale Clinical Scholars Program," which provided "detailed development for the contents of the course, and thereby, for this book" (prologue). This is a scholarly, ambitious text that addresses a multitude of important issues in clinical research design and analysis. Exercises are at the end of each chapter and answers for all chapters follow the final chapter.

Fletcher, R. H.; Fletcher, S. W.; and Wagner, E. H. *Clinical Epidemiology: The Essentials.* 2nd ed., Baltimore: Williams and Wilkins, 1988.

In this new second edition there are no "radical" departures from the characteristics that made the authors' first effort a success. The prose is succinct and major points are clarified with excellent tables and figures. There are two new chapters. The chapter on prevention contains a rather extensive discussion of screening, with many examples. The final chapter, "Summing Up," touches on important aspects of locating and analyzing, individually or as a group, clinical research articles.

Hayden, G. F.; Kramer, M. S.; and Horowitz, R. I. "The Case–Control Study." *JAMA* 247 (1982): 326–31.

This is an extensive review of a common research design. The authors discuss the general structure of research, selection of appropriate case and control groups, definition and detection of the disease under study, and other critical issues in case–control methodology. Two of the authors are pediatricians, and childhood diseases are used for many of the examples.

Henry, R. C.; Massa, M. D., and Ogle, K. S. with Pascoe, J. M., and Singer, D. A. *Planning a Research Study: Pediatric Edition.* East Lansing, Michigan: The Office of Medical Education, Research and Development, 1987.

This packaged workshop and workbook materials are designed to teach new researchers how to design a research plan for their first study. The exercises provide the opportunity for participants to develop hypotheses and operational definitions, a research design, and a timeline and flow chart for research activities. Participants also define outcome measures and establish procedures for data collection using those measures.

Henry, R. C., and Zivick, J. D. "Principles of Survey Research." *Fam Prac Res J* 5 (1986): 145.

An introduction to survey research by explaining 10 basic principles that must be considered when designing surveys. Also includes an item writing checklist for evaluating questionnaire items. The emphasis is on mail questionnaires and includes discussion of sample size, response rates, and formating the survey.

Ibrahim, M. A. *Epidemiology and Health Policy*. Rockville, Maryland: Aspen Publications, 1985.

This book is based on Deon Ibrahim's course on epidemiology and its application to health services and policy. It is succinct, readable, and draws heavily on clinical examples to illustrate basic principles of epidemiology. Major topic areas include epidemiologic foundations of health services, research design and analysis, and preventive services. Chapter 14 specifically addresses several health problems of mothers and children.

Kelsey, J. L.; Thompson, W. D., and Evans, A. S. *Methods in Observational Epidemiology*. New York: Oxford University Press, 1986.

This book may be used as a companion to an introductory textbook on epidemiology or as a resource for those planning epidemiologic research. Although the book focuses on observational or nonexperimental studies, many of the concepts and procedures apply to experimental studies as well. The first three chapters review elementary epidemiologic and biostatistical concepts and methods usually covered in introductory courses. The remaining chapters describe commonly used study designs (e.g., prospective and retrospective cohort studies, cross-sectional and case–control studies). Finally, issues related to measurement, error, and sample size are addressed in detail. There are study exercises but no answers to the questions.

Kleinbaum, D. G.; Kupper, L. L.; and Morgenstern, H. *Epidemiologic Research*. Belmont, California: Wadsworth, 1982.

This text discusses the principles, concepts, and methods involved in the planning analysis, and interpretation of epidemiologic research. The purpose is to provide the reader with a synthesis of methodologic practice and thought. Specifically, the text emphasizes quantitative and statistical issues and therefore may not be ideal for the reader who is seeking an introduction to epidemiology. Nearly 100 pages are devoted to a most helpful discussion of the validity of epidemiologic research. For the more advanced.

Levy, P. A., and Lemeshoe, S. *Sampling for Health Professionals.* Belmont, California: Wadsworth, 1980.

Written for clinical researchers who are experienced in survey design, it also includes many applied techniques and practical examples. The emphasis of the book is on sample design, describing designs ranging from simple to cluster, stratified and stage sampling. It also includes chapters on nonresponse, data collection forms, and interpretation of data for report writing. Practice exercises and a solutions manual are available.

McGaghie, W. C., and Frey, J. J. *Handbook for the Academic Physician.* New York: Springer Verlag, 1986.

This very handy and informative book has six chapters that focus on clinical research. Topics range from a discussion of the role of research in primary care medicine to the specifics of data management. This book is well suited for the beginning researcher who needs guidance in identifying resources to conduct the study and in identifying a plan for managing the study.

Mausner, J. S., and Kramer, S. *Epidemiology: An Introductory Text.* 2nd. ed., Philadelphia: W. B. Saunders, 1985.

The second edition of this introductory text was published 2 years after the death of the first author. It remains an easy-to-read, well-organized introduction to the principles of epidemiology. The 13 chapters describe a number of basic concepts including multiple causation of disease, rates, ratios and proportions, screening, and types of analytic studies.

Marks, R. G. *Designing a Research Project.* Belmont, California: Wadsworth, 1982.

This book teaches the basic concepts of research design through a step-by-step guide. It explains how to determine project objectives, deciding what type of data to collect, and how to design a data collection form. Two chapters that are very practical describe how to determine the proper sample size for the study.

Nieme, R. G., and Sullivan, J. L., eds. *Quantitative Applications in the Social Science.* Beverly Hills: Sage Publications, 1976–

Although written for social scientists, the Sage Publications are practical and inexpensive papers that are designed to improve the methodological skills of all researchers. There are now 60 papers in this series that focus on a variety of research topics for the beginner and the advanced researcher. The papers are clearly written and are as useful for the primary care researcher as they are the social scientist. A sampling of titles: Tests of Significance; Analysis of Variance; Analysis of Nominal and Ordinal Data; Factor Analysis; Measures of Association; Survey Sampling. For a complete listing of titles and descriptions write the publisher: P.O. Box 5024, Beverly Hills, California 90210, (213) 274-8003.

Statistics

Bailer, J. C., and Mosteller, F. *Medical Uses of Statistics.* Waltham, Massachusetts: NEJM Books, 1986.

> Another "second level" book on statistics, "This book surveys the state of the art statistical applications in clinical research and illustrates good and poor uses of methods" (Introduction). Thirteen of the 20 chapters are originally published in the *New England Journal of Medicine* between 1983 and 1985. While this text draws heavily on clinical examples, there are no exercises to facilitate the reader's exploration of "good and poor uses of methods."
>
> Since 1980 George W. Brown, M.D. has published a number of well-written articles that explain many of the major issues in clinical research. The relevance of his papers is enhanced by the fact that most of the examples are taken from the practice of pediatric medicine. It is believed that they have not been published in monograph form. The citations in Chronological order are as follows:

Brown, G. W. "Regression and Clinical Research." *Am J Dis Child* 134 (1980); 549–52.
———. "Bayes' Formula: Conditional Probability and Clinical Medicine." *Am J Dis Child* 135 (1981): 1125–29.
———. "Standard Deviation, Standard Error: Which 'Standard' Should We Use?" *Am J Dis Child* 136 (1982): 937–41.
———. "Errors, Types I and II." *Am J Dis Child* 137 (1983): 586–91.
———. "Discriminant Analysis." *Am J Dis Child* 138 (1984): 395–400.
———. "Counts, Scales and Scores." *Am J Dis Child* 139 (1985): 147–51.
———. "Statistics and the Medical Journal." (editorial), *Am J Dis Child* 139 (1985): 226–28.

———. "2 × 2 Tables." *Am J Dis Child* 139 (1985): 410–16.

——— and Baca, G. M. "A Classification of Original Articles. American Journal of Diseases of Children 1983 and 1984." *Am J Dis Child* 140 (1986): 641–45.

——— and Hayden, G. F. "Nonparametric Methods: Clinical Applications." *Clin Pediatr* 24 (1985): 490–98.

Colton, T. *Statistics in Medicine*. Boston: Little, Brown and Company, 1982.

> This book examines statistical principles from the view of the research consumer, the reader. The book is divided into three divisions. Part I introduces basic concepts, definitions and principles of descriptive statistics and probability. Part II builds a foundation for understanding statistical inference; drawing conclusions about populations based on data from samples. The chapters cover all the frequently used statistical tests encountered in the general medical literature. Part III discusses the use of statistics in medical research and contains chapters on clinical trials, medical surveys, and identifies common pitfalls when drawing conclusions from medical research.

Kleinbaum, D. G., and Kupper, L. L. *Applied Regression Analysis and Other Multivariate Methods*. North Scituate, Massachusetts: Duxbury Press, 1978.

> This "second level" biostatistics text is dedicated to the late epidemiologist John C. Cassel. It is based on a biostatistics course designed for nonstatistics majors in health and related fields. Early chapters address the choice of analysis and a review of basic statistics. Regression, correlation, analysis of variance, factor analysis, discriminant analysis, and the linear models approach to the analysis of categorical data are discussed in a readable fashion. The text is filled with examples and there are exercises (with answers) at the end of each chapter.

Kramer, H. C., and Thiemann, S. *How Many Subjects? Statistical Power Analysis in Research*. Newbury Park, California: Sage Publications, 1987.

> A practical "how-to" book that explains not only how to determine sample size but also offers useful principles for cost-effective research. It is written in clear and simple language so the begin-

ning researcher should have little difficulty following the computational steps for the type of study design selected.

Marks, E. G. *Analyzing Research Data: The Basics of Biomedical Research Methodology.* Belmont, California: Wadsworth, 1982.

This book teaches fundamental statistical techniques used in analyzing and evaluating clinical data. Emphasis is on selection of the appropriate statistical analysis and interpretation of data from computer printouts. While not as comprehensive as some texts, it does focus on essential techniques such as the Z tests, ANOVA, nonparametric techniques, discriminant analysis, and time series. These companion books assume no previous knowledge of statistics and design issues.

These two books are companions and a must for the beginning researcher. The author is both a teacher of research methodology and a researcher himself. This is evident to the reader who receives a logical and very organized approach to research design and data analysis.

Norman, G. R., and Streinder, D. L. *PDQ Statistics.* Burlington, Ontario: B.C. Decker, 1986.

This book is both fun and informative yet covers a wide range of topics from simple t tests to multivariate and advanced nonparametric methods. The explanations and medical examples are simple to follow. The purpose of the book is to assist the reader in understanding the results section of a research article and not to compute actual statistics. This book might best be used in conjunction with an introductory statistics textbook.

O'Brien, P. C., and Shampo, M. A. "Statistics for Clinicians." *Mayo Clin Proc* 56 (1981): 45–6.

A reprint series available from the journal. A most practical overview of descriptive and inferential statistical techniques used in clinical research. The writing is nontechnical and very appropriate for the beginning researcher. In all there are 12 nontechnical papers that briefly address the following topics in statistics: descriptive statistics; graphic displays; estimation from samples; one and two sample t test; regression; chi-square and the relative deviate test; evaluating diagnostic procedures; normal values; survivorship studies; and sequential methods.

Schefler, W. C. *Statistics for Health Professionals.* Reading, Massachusetts: Addison-Wesley Publishing Company, 1984.

> A good introduction to statistics that does not assume any mathematics beyond high school algebra. The emphasis is placed on applied statistics as a set of principles and a way of thinking rather than a series of exercises in mathematics. The chapter on probability is especially well written in that it incorporates many examples from specific diseases that are common to clinical medicine. Similar to other introductory textbooks, there are chapters on comparing means; proportions; regression analysis; correlations; and analysis of covariance. The new researcher may find this to be one of the most readable texts on statistics.

Young, M. J.; Bresnit, E. A.; and Strom, B. L. Sample Size Nomogram for Interpreting Negative Clinical Studies. *Ann Intern Med* 99 (1983): 248.

> The big question for many researchers is, How many subjects do I need? (the nomogram) This brief article provides a useful strategy for nomogram interpreting negative studies and also for determining sample size for projected studies. A practice example is included for readers to apply the nomogram to a real research situation.

Clinical Research Funding

The Foundation Directory. New York: The Foundation Center, 1984.

> This directory lists nearly all foundations that support research and scholarship. The directory provides listings by state and subject area. A brief description of funding history is also included.

NIH Guide for Grants and Contracts. Bethesda: U.S. Department of Health and Human Services, 15 (2): 1986.

> This guide published several times a year announces new and continuing grant programs of the NIH. Useful resource for researchers.

Update on the Catalog of Federal Domestic Assistance 1986. Washington
D.C.: Government Printing Office, 1986.

> Lists all programs funded by the federal government. Because of
> extensive documentation, this is a difficult resource to use effi-
> ciently.

Related and Interesting

Kuhn, T. *The Structure of Scientific Revolutions.* Chicago: University of
Chicago Press, 1964.

> An excellent discussion of how science develops and how scien-
> tific paradigms are accepted and rejected throughout time. Kuhn
> takes a historical perspective by charting the nature of "normal
> science" and then describes how scientific discoveries occur
> through anomalies and crises. The final chapters address the
> necessity of scientific revolution and the progress made by them.
> This book works well for a seminar on the history or philosophy
> of science. A classic that any serious researcher should read.

9

Glossary

ALAIN JOFFE

Attack Rate: The percent of exposed susceptible individuals developing a disease or symptom during a specified time period. For example, if 20 of 100 nonimmune individuals exposed to rubella virus develop rubella, the attack rate is 20 percent.

Bias: A systematic error in study design or in inference from study data such that the study results differ from true values. Bias can be introduced at any point in the study design, execution, or interpretation.

Case–control study: A retrospective observational study design that begins with identification of subjects with (cases) and without (controls) an outcome of interest. The cases and controls are then evaluated for prior exposures to risk factors of interest.

Cluster Sampling: Random probability samples of aggregates of subjects rather than individual subjects.

Concurrent study: A prospective study in which the researcher and subjects move forward together in time from the point of exposure or initiation of study.

Confidence intervals (usually expressed as 95 percent confidence interval or CI): the range of possible results around the study result based on study design and sample size. For example, if a study showed a 20 percent reduction in blood pressure after salt restriction, the 95 percent CI might be 6–34 percent reduction based on a given sample size.

Confounding: A possible source of bias in comparative studies in that an unmeasured third variable (the confounder) is (1) associated with the exposure of interest and (2) causally related to the outcome of interest.

Content validity: The extent to which items in a measure (instrument) actually reflect the full range or domain of the concept the investigator wishes to measure or assess.

Continuous data: Data to which numbers are assigned or attached that have absolute meaning (e.g., age, height, weight, scores on the MCATS).

Convenience sampling: A nonprobability method of sampling in which the most readily available subjects of interest are chosen without regard to potential bias.

Correlation coefficient: A measure of association indicating the strength and direction of the relationship between two variables.

Criterion validity: The ability of one measure (instrument) to predict performance on another measure of the same construct. For example, the ability of the 4-question CAGE alcoholism screening test to predict performance on the 25-question MAST alcoholism screening test.

Cross-sectional study: A study designed to document relationships between two or more groups or among various attributes of a single group at a single point in time. Also called prevalence studies.

Dependent variable (*criterion measure*): The result (outcome) under study as being affected by various factors. For example, in studying the effect of salt restriction on blood pressure, blood pressure (or changes in blood pressure) is the dependent variable.

Ecologic fallacy: Descriptive data gathered at a group level applied erroneously to a single individual or small subset of that group.

External validity: The extent to which study results can be extrapolated or generalized beyond the study population and setting. Also referred to as a study's clinical usefulness.

Hypothesis: A precise, testable statement of a research question. A *null* hypothesis predicts no difference will be discovered between the groups to be studied. A *directional* hypothesis predicts that a difference will exist and in which direction.

Independent variable(s): A factor that may cause an effect on the outcome to be studied (the *dependent* variable). For example, in studying the effect of maternal age on the percent of infants riding in car seats, maternal age is the *independent* variable.

Informed consent: A principle governing research on human subjects. It expresses the ideal that research subjects voluntarily agree to participate in research protocols based on a clear understanding of the project and the benefits and risks accruing to him or her from participation in the study.

Internal consistency: Refers to the concept that when using a multi-item scale or instrument to measure a construct, *each* of the items should be measuring the same thing. Usually reported in terms of *Cronbach's alpha*.

Internal validity: Refers to the statistical and methodologic rigor of a study design so as to eliminate uncontrolled influences that could bias study results.

Matching: The creation of comparable study groups through the selection of subjects on the basis of certain key variables (e.g., race, age, sex, socioeconomic status).

Mean value: The average value of all data points, calculated from the sum of individual values divided by the total number of measurements.

Median value: The value that separates all the data points into halves. Fifty percent of the points are below the median and 50 percent above. Usually applied to ordinal variables.

Mode: The value that occurs most frequently in the data set.

Nominal data: Data that are classified unordered into categories (e.g., race, sex, country of origin).

Nonconcurrent study: A prospective observational study design that begins with individuals exposed or not exposed to a risk factor at a point in the past and then followed forward in time to study the relation between an outcome of interest and the risk factor of interest.

Nonprobability sampling: The method of sampling whereby no estimation of the probability of including any given individual from a population in a study sample is possible.

Ordinal data: Data that are logically ordered in nature (1+, 2+, 3+ pitting edema, small, medium, large body frame). A categorical type of data.

Predictive value of a negative test:
$$\frac{\text{True negative}}{\text{True negative} + \text{False negative}} \quad \text{(Expressed as \%)} \quad .$$

Predictive value of a positive test:
$$\frac{\text{True positives}}{\text{True positives} + \text{False positives}} \quad \text{(Expressed as \%)} \quad .$$

Probability sampling: The method of sampling whereby one can specify for each person in the population, the probability that he or she will be included in the sample.

Prospective study: A study design in which groups of subjects are identified at the time of an exposure or event and followed forward in time to determine an outcome.

Purposive sampling: A nonprobability method of sampling in which the investigator assumes that a representative sample can be chosen based on good judgment and/or appropriate strategies.

Random allocation: The method of assigning individuals to control and experimental groups such that each subject has an equal chance of being assigned to any of the groups.

Regression to the mean: Refers to the concept that individuals (or subjects) chosen by virtue of extreme values (e.g., low test scores) can in effect change in only one direction under experimental conditions. Hence, the change is erroneously attributed to the intervention under study.

Reliability: Refers to the consistency of repeated measurements (observations, etc.) across subjects or between observers; a reflection of measurement error. Reliable measurements reflect true differences as opposed to instability of the device or observer. More reliable measures produce results that cluster closely around the true value.

Sample: The proportion of the population at large to be studied. When used as a verb (to sample; sampling), it refers to the process of subject selection.

Sensitivity: $$\frac{\text{True positives}}{\text{True positives} + \text{False negatives}}$$ (Expressed as %)

Simple random sampling: The most basic probability sampling method. Each element in the population has an equal chance of being included in the study sample.

Specificity: $$\frac{\text{True negatives}}{\text{True negatives} + \text{False positives}}$$ (Expressed as %)

Statistical power: The ability of a study of given size to detect a true difference. More powerful studies are able to detect smaller differences.

Stratified random sampling: Simple random samples selected from subcategories of a population (e.g., men, women, blacks, Hispanics).

Systematic sampling: A probability sampling method in which every *n*th case is chosen from a population in which all subjects have been assigned consecutive numbers.

Type I error: In hypothesis testing, refers to the situation in which a statistically significant association is discovered when in reality no such association exists.

Type II error: Failure to detect (at a statistically significant level) a difference between two or more groups when in reality a difference exists.

Validity: Refers to the concept that the study (a valid study) demonstrates what actually exists or that the measure (a valid measure) actually assesses what the investigator intends.

Index

Abstracts, writing, 107
Aggregate data, 77
Alpha value, 99
Altemeir, W. A., 59
Alternative hypothesis, 18
American Medical Association, 23
Analysis of variance (ANOVA), 101
Annals of Internal Medicine, The, xv, 64
Annual Register of Grant Support, 124
Attack rate, 155
Attrition of study subjects, 34–35

Baseline percentage, 32
Bias, 155
  in availability of patients, 51
  referral, 136
Bibliography, annotated, 144–154
Biostatistician, working with, 7, 16, 106
Budgeting, *see* Costs

Campbell, D. T., 11, 60, 66–68, 69
Case-control studies, 35, 40, 56–58, 155
Case findings, 142
Catalog of Federal Domestic Assistance, 124
Categorical variables, 97
Causal inference, 7–8
Cause–effect relationship, strength of support for, 42–43, 44
Chi-square test, 101, 103
Circular concept in research development, 20

Clinical journal articles, critical appraisal of, 133–143
  on diagnosis, 136–137
  on etiology or causation of disease, 134–136
  on prognosis, 137–138
  on screening, 141–143
  on therapy, 139–140
Clinical Research Center (CRC) programs, 119
Clinical trials, 62–72
Clinical Trials (Meinert), 65
Cluster sampling, 28, 29, 155
CME programs (medical news service), 23
Code of Federal Regulations of Department of Health and Human Services, 126–131
Coding manual, 91
Cohort studies, observational, 40–41, 59–62
Collaboration, 132
Commerce Business Daily, 124
Communication of results, *see* Data reporting
Community foundations, 121
Compatability (computer compatability), 93–94
Comparative studies, 35–37, 56–72
  case-control studies, 35, 40, 56–58, 155
  descriptive studies versus, 47–48
  experimental studies, 41, 62–72
  matching, 36–37

Comparative studies (*continued*)
  observational cohort studies, 40–41, 59–62
  observational studies, 56–62
  quasi-experimental studies, 41, 66–72
  random allocation, 35–36, 158
Computer-based directories of funding sources, 123
Concurrent studies, 44–46, 155
Confidence interval, 103–104, 155–156
Confounding variables, 96, 102, 156
Construct, 80–81
  inference to, 9–10
Construct validity, 12, 84
Consultants, 20–21
Content validity (face validity), 81, 156
Continuous data, 76, 156
Continuous variables, 96
Contracts, 117, 121
Control group, 19
Control variables, 96
Convenience (accidental) sampling, 28, 156
Cook, T. D., 11
Cooperative agreement, 118
Corporate foundations, 121
Correlation coefficient, 99–100, 156
Costs
  categories of expense and level of detail required in budget proposal, 113
  minimizing, 114–115
  projecting, 112–114
Criterion measure (dependent variable), 19
Criterion validity, 81–82, 156
Cronbach's alpha, 84, 157
Cross-over studies, 66
Cross-sectional studies, 52–56, 156
Crosstabulations, 98

Data analysis, xiv–xv, 3, 94–106
  alternatives to significance testing, 103–104
  common pitfalls, 105
  initial descriptive analysis, 96–99
  overview of, 95–96
  statistical tests of significance, 99–103
  working with a statistician, 106
Data-base management, 22–23, 92
Data collection, xiii–xiv, 3, 75–89
  information requirements, 75–77
  minimizing costs, 114–115
  selecting collection instrument or measures, 78–89
  sources of available data, 77–78
Data entry, 91–94
Data management procedures, 89–94
  coding manual, 91
  data entry, 91–94
  procedures manual, 89–90
Data reporting, xv–xvi, 106–110
  presentations, 107–108
  publication, 108–110
  writing an abstract, 107
Dependent variable (criterion measure), 18, 96, 156
Descriptive analysis, initial, 96–99
Descriptive studies, 49–52
  comparative studies versus, 47–48
Diagnostic tests for causation, 44
DIALOG (data-base system), 23
Directional hypothesis, 156
Discrete variables, 96
Documentation of procedures, *see* Procedures manual
Donation, 118
Drug industry, funding support by, 120

Ecologic fallacy, 77, 156
Ecologic studies, 52–56
Eligible subjects, systematic search for, 50
Ellenberg, J. H., 51
Epidemiologic cohorts, 60
Errors, types I and II, 99, 159
Ethical standards for research involving human subjects, 126–131

Experimental studies, 41, 62–72
  observational studies versus, 48–49
External validity, 12, 156

Factors, 17
Family foundations, 121
Federal Register, 124
Feinstein, A. R., 49–50, 58, 62, 64, 68
Fellowship, 118
FIRST (First Independent Research
    Support and Transition) award,
    118, 122
Fisher's exact test, 101, 103
Form PHS 398 (application for Public
    Health Service Grant), 125
Foundation Directory, The, 124
Foundation Grant Index, The, 124
Foundation grants, 120–121
Frequency matching, 36–37
Funding, 112, 115–116
  applying for research support, 123–
    126
  guidelines for, 116
  identifying potential sources of, 121–
    123, 124–125
  private sources, 120–121
  public sources, 119
  sources of, 116–118

Generalizability, 10
Gift, 118
Glossary, 155–159
Gould, Stephen J., 85
Grants, 117–118, 121
  foundation, 120–121
Guyatt, G., 70

Herford, Oliver, xvi
Human subjects, ethical standards for
    research involving, 126–131
Hypothesis, 156
  definition of, 17
  two basic types of, 18
Hypothesis formation, 17–18
Hypothesis testing, 17

Illinois Researcher Information System
    (IRIS), 123
Independent variables, 19–20, 96, 157
Index Medicus, The, 21
Inference, 4–5
  causal, 7–8
  statistical, 5–7, 94
Informed consent, 157
  general requirement for,
    130–131
In-house research seminars, 16
Initial descriptive analysis, 96–99
Institutional human investigation
    review board, 16
Internal consistency, 84, 157
Internal validity, 12, 157
Interrater reliability, 88
Intrarater reliability, 87

Lilienfeld, A. M., 54, 58
Literature search, 21–24
Louis, T. A., 66

Matching, 36–37, 157
Mean, 97, 98, 157
Mean matching, 36, 37
Measures, 18–20
  modification of, 88–89
Median, 97, 98, 157
MEDIS (medical full-text service), 23
MEDLARS (Medical Literature
    Analysis and Retrieval System), 22
MEDLINE (data-base system), 22, 23
Meinert, C. L., 65
Meta-analysis, 43
Microcomputer for data entry, 91–94
Mode, 97, 98, 157
Modification of the measure, 88–89
Multiple regression analysis, 102
Multivariant discriminant analysis, 102

National foundations, 120
National Library of Medicine, 23
National Library of Medicine
    Bibliography, 21

National Science Foundation Guide to Programs, 125
Nelson, K. B., 51
NIH Guide to Grants and Contracts, 118, 122, 124
Nominal data, 76, 95–96, 157
Nonconcurrent studies, 44–46, 157
Nonequivalent control group design, 68–69
Nonpair matching, 36–37
Nonparametric tests, 102–103
Nonprobability sampling, 25, 26, 28–31, 157
  combination of probability sampling and, 31
  convenience sampling, 28, 156
  purposive sampling, 30, 158
  quota sampling, 30
  special applications of, 30–31
Null hypothesis, 18, 156
Numerical variables, 96, 97–98

Observational cohort studies, 40–41, 59–62
Observational studies, 56–62
  experimental studies versus, 48–49
Observations, classifying, rules for, 51–52
Observed group, criteria for inclusion in, 50
Odds ratio, 104
Ordinal data, 76, 157
Ordinal variables, 96
Orientation of the study in time, 43–46
Outcome percentage, 32
Outliers, 96–97

Packet switching networks, 22
Paired *t*-test, 101
Pair matching, 36
Paperchase (data-base system), 23
Parametric tests, 100
Patients, assessment of bias in availability of, 51
Place factors, 17

Predictive value of a negative test, 158
Predictive value of a positive test, 158
Presentation of a study, 107–108
Primary data, 77
Private funding sources, 120–121
Probability sampling, 25, 26–28, 158
  cluster sampling, 28, 29, 155
  combination of nonprobability sampling and, 31
  simple random sampling, 26–27, 159
  stratified random sampling, 27–28, 159
  systematic sampling, 27, 159
Probability value (*p* value), 99
Procedures manual, 89–90
Programmatic data, 77
Prospective (longitudinal) study, 59, 158
  retrospective study versus, 46–47
Publication, 108–110
Public funding sources, 119
Public Health Service Act, 126
Purely descriptive cohort study, 60
Purposive sampling, 30, 158

Quasi-experimental studies, 41, 66–72
  intransigency situation number one, 68–69
  intransigency situation number two, 69
  intransigency situation number three, 70–72
Question (research question), xi–xiii, 14–20
  factors to be measured, 19–20
  forming the hypothesis, 17–18
  generating creative ideas, 16
  identifying a simple question, 16–17
  modifying the question, 17
Quota sampling, 30

Random allocation, 35–36, 158
Random sampling
  simple, 26–27, 159
  stratified, 27–28, 159
Range, 98

"Ranked" correlation test (Kendall's or Spearman's correlation), 101, 103
Ranked variables, 96
Reading a medical journal article, *see* Clinical journal article, critical appraisal of
Referral bias, 136
Regression to the mean, 47, 158
Relative odds, 58
Reliability, 86–88, 158
Remedial trials, 62–63
Request for Applications (RFA), 121–122
Research, steps in, xii
Research Awards Index, 125
Research clubs, 16
Research models and methods, 38–74
    choosing a study design, 39–49
    classifications of study design, 38–39, 40–41
    comparative studies, 56–72
    cross-sectional and ecologic studies, 52–56
    descriptive studies, 49–52
    key aspects of, 3
Retrospective studies, prospective studies versus, 46–47
Risk ratio, 104
Routine data, 77
Rules for classifying observations, 51–52

Sackett, D. L., 52, 58, 61
Sample, 25–26, 158
Sample size, 31–34
Sampling
    nonprobability, 25, 26, 28–31, 157
    probability, 25, 26–28, 158
Scattergrams, 98–99
Schneeweiss, R., 52
SCISEARCH (data-base system), 23
Sensitivity, 158
Simple random sampling, 26–27, 159
Single heterogeneous group, 59
Special interest foundations, 120–121

Specificity, 159
Sponsored Programs Information Network (SPIN), 123
Spread-sheet program, 92
Standard deviation, 98
Stanley, J. C., 60, 66–68, 69
Statistical consultation, 21
Statistical inference, 5–7, 94
Statistical Package for the Social Sciences (SPSS), 84–85
Statistical packages, 93
Statistical power, 159
Statistical tests of significance, 99–103
Statistical validity, 11–12
Statisticians, working with, 7, 16, 106
Steinwachs, D. M., 52
Steps in clinical research, xii
Stratification, 102
Stratified random sampling, 27–28, 159
Study design, 3, 4
    choosing, 39–49
    classifications of, 38–39, 40–41
    five considerations for, xi–xvi
Subcontractors, use of, 114
Subjects for study, xiii, 25–37
    attrition of subjects, 34–35
    combination of probability and nonprobability samples, 31
    comparative studies, 35–37
    eligible, systematic search for, 50
    nonprobability sampling techniques, 25, 26, 28–31, 157
    probability sampling techniques, 25, 26–28, 158
    sample selections, 3, 25–26
    sample size, 31–34
    See also Human subjects
Systematic sampling, 27, 159

Test group, 19
Time, xvi–xvii, 17
    orientation of the study in, 43–46

Time-series analysis, 70–71
t-test, 100, 101
Two homogeneous groups, 60
Type I error, 99, 159
Type II error, 99, 159

Validity, 11–12, 80–86, 159
  construct, 12, 84
  content (face), 81, 156
  criterion, 81–82, 156
  external, 12, 156
  internal, 12, 157
  statistical, 11–12
Variables, 3, 95–96

  categorical, 97
  confounding, 96, 102, 156
  continuous, 96
  control, 96
  dependent, 18, 96, 156
  discrete, 96
  independent, 19–20, 96, 157
  numerical, 96, 97–98
  ordinal, 96
  ranked, 96
Variance, 98

Word-processing programs, 92–93
Writing an abstract, 107